The Condensed Curriculum Guide

The Condensed Curriculum

FOR GP TRAINING AND THE NEW MRCGP

BEN RILEY, JAYNE HAYNES AND STEVE FIELD

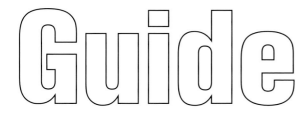

Guide

Royal College of
General Practitioners

The Royal College of General Practitioners was founded
in 1952 with this object:

'*To encourage, foster and maintain the highest possible standards
in general practice and for that purpose to take or join with others
in taking steps consistent with the charitable nature of that object
which may assist towards the same.*'

Among its responsibilities under its Royal Charter the
College is entitled to:

'*Diffuse information on all matters affecting general practice and
issue such publications as may assist the object of the College.*'

British Library Cataloguing-in-Publication Data
A catalogue record for this book is available from the British Library

© Royal College of General Practitioners, 2007
Published by the Royal College of General Practitioners, 2007
14 Princes Gate, Hyde Park, London SW7 1PU

Disclaimer
This publication is intended for the use of medical practitioners in the UK
and not for patients. The authors, editors and publisher have taken care to
ensure that the information contained in this book is correct to the best of their
knowledge, at the time of publication. Whilst efforts have been made to ensure
the accuracy of the information presented, particularly that related to the
prescription of drugs, the authors, editors and publisher cannot accept liability
for information that is subsequently shown to be wrong. Readers are advised
to check that the information, especially that related to drug usage, complies
with information contained in the *British National Formulary,* or equivalent,
or manufacturers' datasheets, and that it complies with the latest legislation
and standards of practice.

Designed and typeset at the Typographic Design Unit

Printed by Cromwell Press Group

Indexed by Carol Ball

ISBN 978-0-85084-316-3

Dedication

This book is dedicated to all the team members at Poplar Grove Practice, Aylesbury, and 19 Beaumont Street Surgery, Oxford– your positive influence on our first experience of general practice shaped much of the advice contained in this guide.

Contents

About the authors

Dr Ben Riley MRCGP is a practising GP in Faringdon, in rural Oxfordshire. As RCGP Curriculum Development Fellow, he is responsible for the ongoing development of educational resources to support GPs in training. He completed his own GP training on the Aylesbury Vocational Training Scheme in 2004, having gained his MRCGP with distinction. He has written about the reality of being a GP trainee in a number of publications and completed a Masters-level evaluation of his early experiences of learning in general practice to obtain his Postgraduate Certificate in Primary Care.

Dr Jayne Haynes MRCGP is a practising GP in a well-established training practice in the city centre of Oxford. She undertook her GP training on the Oxford Vocational Training Scheme, where she gained her MRCGP with distinction, before taking a senior registrar post in academic general practice. After working for a short spell in New Zealand, she returned to her former training practice in Oxford, where she is involved in the education of specialty registrars (GP). She enjoys being a 'generalist' and has particular interests in general medicine and student health.

Professor Steve Field FRCGP has been elected as the Chairman of the Royal College of General Practitioners from November 2007. As leader of the RCGP's Professional Development Board, he spearheaded the introduction of the RCGP Curriculum for Specialty Training for General Practice. Steve is a practising GP in inner-city Birmingham, the Regional Postgraduate Dean for West Midlands Deanery and a member of the Postgraduate Medical Education and Training Board (PMETB). He is also Honorary Professor of Medical Education at the University of Warwick and an Honorary Professor of the School of Medicine at the University of Birmingham. He has published many academic papers on general practice and a range of books on GP education and training.

Foreword

Isn't it strange? If you meet someone socially for the first time and tell them you are a doctor, there is an awful inevitability about what they will say next – 'Are you a specialist or just a GP?' It is that use of the word 'just' that causes the heart to sink – probably in the same way that patients feel their hearts sink when we say their condition is 'just a virus'.

But being a GP is hugely complex. There is something breathtakingly illogical about the way that society generally bestows the highest prestige on those whose area of expertise is smallest, and vice versa. But the undeniable truth is that being a GP is an extraordinarily complex task. After all, patients can, and do, bring us problems of every imaginable dimension, and expect us to have an answer.

The RCGP's magnificent new curriculum for GP training demonstrates the enormity of the task facing family doctors. No one will ever again be able to describe general practice as the simple option, but demonstrating this complexity brings its own problems. Faced with the whole curriculum, many doctors might think they need a simpler career choice – like cardio-thoracic surgery.

And so a book like this is invaluable. This book has two main purposes: it makes the curriculum accessible by condensing it into its core educational material, and it provides practical guidance both on how to learn and how to teach it. Whilst primarily aimed at trainees, parts are of real value to GP educators as well. The authors have deliberately tried to keep the approach pragmatic and point readers towards useful sources of information or practical approaches to learning.

The first half of the book is called 'The Curriculum Guide' and it contains chapters on the background and development of the curriculum, how it is organised, how to learn and teach it, and how to prepare for the new MRCGP assessments. The second part is 'The Condensed Curriculum' and contains the chapters describing and interpreting the first curriculum statement, *Being a General Practitioner*, which explores the core competences of general practice.

General practice needs this book. But, much more importantly and indirectly, so do our patients. After all, high-quality general practice is of vital importance to patients everywhere. GPs really do make a difference.

Professor David Haslam CBE, FRCP, FFPH, PRCGP
President, Royal College of General Practitioners

Acknowledgements

We would like to thank the many people involved in the RCGP curriculum project whose effort provided the groundwork for this book. In particular, we would like to thank Mike Deighan for his dedicated and irreplaceable contribution.

We would also like to express our gratitude to our former trainers, Martin Wakeford and Meriel Raine, for the invaluable support and advice they provided during our GP training, and to Marion Lynch for opening the door to the wider world of adult education and making this book possible.

What's in this guide?

Part III: Appendices and index

Part I

The curriculum guide

1 Introducing the curriculum

What is the RCGP curriculum?

The RCGP Curriculum for Specialty Training for General Practice has been developed to guide doctors through their three-year period of specialist training for general practice. It is an educational document designed to help learners develop the wide-ranging knowledge, clinical skills, communication techniques and professional attitudes considered essential for a doctor practising in primary care in the modern UK National Health Service.

This chapter explains some of the background to how the new curriculum came into existence and will help you understand what the curriculum is all about.

Is it meant for me?

The curriculum has been designed for four main groups.

First and foremost, the curriculum is intended to meet the educational needs of GPs in training.[i] For the first time ever, it presents an official view of the core knowledge, skills, attitudes and expertise that a doctor needs to learn and develop to become a competent GP. It takes the broad principles of the General Medical Council's *Good Medical Practice* document,[1] and applies them directly to everyday general practice.

Secondly, the curriculum is a useful guide for GP educators. It forms a framework for trainers, course organisers and other GP educators to plan their training and mentoring, and to design their local educational programmes.

Thirdly, the curriculum has been designed to meet the needs of the Postgraduate Medical Education and Training Board (PMETB),[2] the regulatory authority with responsibility for general practice training in the UK. The clear standards of competence described in the curriculum are important for promoting public confidence in the quality of general practice as a profession. The curriculum is designed to form a reliable benchmark against which the performance of new GPs can be assessed at the end of their training, and also to inform the design of the assessments that will be used in the revalidation of established GPs.

Fourthly, the curriculum is intended for academic GPs and for those interested in educational research and the development of GP training. The curriculum describes an evidence-based view of

---

[i] GPs in training are officially referred to as specialty registrars (GP).

contemporary general practice and will aid the continuing development of general practice as a generalist medical specialty.

The evolution of the curriculum

The curriculum was developed over three years with input from a broad range of people and organisations.

To begin the process, two 'curriculum working groups' were set up by the Education Department of the Royal College of General Practitioners. One was asked to deal with Learning and Teaching and the other with Assessment. Each group had representatives from a variety of backgrounds, including working GPs, trainers, other primary-care educators, secondary-care experts, GP trainees and members of the public.

A strong evidence-based approach was taken to the development of the curriculum. A literature review was commissioned from the Centre for Research in Medical and Dental Education at the University of Birmingham, who have published widely in this area.[3] At the same time, an extensive consultation exercise was carried out, which included:

- A national questionnaire survey of the views of trainees and GP educators

- Meetings with patient representatives, members of the public and GP trainees

- Focus groups and presentations at national and international conferences on GP education to share findings and explore ideas.

After this process was complete, the first curriculum statement was written: *Being a General Practitioner*. This formed the template for the other 31 statements that make up the curriculum. Each statement was coordinated by a GP with particular expertise in that particular field. The statements were then circulated in draft form to GPs, educators, patient representatives, members of the public, trainees and specialist interest groups within the RCGP. They were also posted on the RCGP website. There was a period of formal consultation and revision before finally the whole bundle of statements was submitted to PMETB (the regulatory body) for approval.

Keeping the curriculum up-to-date

General practice is a constantly changing profession and the curriculum must be adaptable to the ever-changing circumstances in primary care, such as changes that come about as a result of new government policy or unexpected national events.

Each statement in the curriculum has a named 'guardian'. Guardians are responsible for the monitoring of their statement and for proposing any changes to the RCGP's Education Network. Each statement in the curriculum is reviewed annually and rewritten every five years, and this process is being staged so that each year about six statements undergo a rewrite. After six years, once every statement has been through one full cycle of review, the curriculum as a whole will be reviewed. This whole process is known as a 'root and branch' review.

GP training in the UK is organised by local regions, known as deaneries. Each deanery will collect a range of data every year to feed into the curriculum review process. These will include quality assurance reports, GP trainee performance data, national exit survey data and the views of local educators in the deanery.

GP educators, trainees, members of the public and patients will continue to remain involved in the ongoing monitoring of the curriculum. All specialty registrars will complete an exit survey on the completion of their training and both trainees and patient representatives will be included in the five-yearly review process for each statement.

The role of the curriculum in GP training

The curriculum describes the core competences that a GP is expected to master by the end of the three-year training programme. This should mean that the days are gone when a new GP trainee spends weeks searching fruitlessly for an official opinion on 'what a GP needs to know'. GPs in training can now focus their efforts instead on developing the identified core knowledge, attitudes and skills of general practice. The curriculum also contains a useful syllabus of key knowledge that will be used as a basis for the nMRCGP assessments, in particular the Applied Knowledge Test examination.

How the curriculum is applied to individual learners will vary considerably from person to person, and it is extremely important for GPs in training to develop their adult learning skills and to identify their individual learning needs.

As well as being particularly useful for current trainees and their educational supervisors, the curriculum is relevant to a much wider group of people. The curriculum has a role to play for every GP who is actively wishing to maintain good standards of professional practice – providing a blueprint for continuing professional development (CPD) and lifelong medical education.

How GP training is organised

The GP Specialty Training Programme, which is covered by the curriculum, runs for three years from the end of the two-year Foundation Programme to the award of the Certificate of Completion of Training, when a doctor qualifies as a GP. During this time, GPs in training are officially referred to as GP specialty registrars.

Applications for places on GP training programmes are processed through a national selection scheme. Each training programme has a Programme Director, who has responsibility for the sequence of posts that make up the programme and the quality of the training that is provided. Educators based in primary care and secondary care help directors to deliver the training. The emphasis continues to be on learning in the workplace although some teaching is arranged more formally with courses and day-release programmes, including a number of mandatory courses (e.g. child protection). Ongoing mentoring and educational supervision will take place throughout the three years.

Figure 1.1

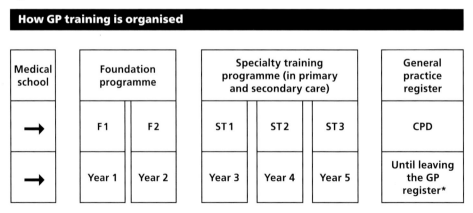

How GP training is organised

Medical school	Foundation programme		Specialty training programme (in primary and secondary care)			General practice register
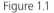	F1	F2	ST1	ST2	ST3	CPD
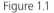	Year 1	Year 2	Year 3	Year 4	Year 5	Until leaving the GP register*

F = foundation   ST = specialty training   CPD = Continuing Professional Development
*usually at retirement age, unless you are lucky enough to win the lottery!

How to use the curriculum in everyday general practice

This is why we have written this guide.

At first glance, the biggest difficulty with using the curriculum is its enormous size and extremely broad coverage. The 32 statements contain over 500 pages and around 1350 learning outcomes, and a full printout weighs about 3·5 kg! However, once you start to examine the curriculum more closely, you will discover it is not quite as vast or inaccessible as it may at first seem.

You will have noticed that this guide is a fraction of the size of the full curriculum. So how it is possible to compress a comprehensive 500 page document into a single volume? This is explained in the following chapter, which describes how the curriculum itself is organised and what the fancy educational words like 'competency' and 'learning outcome' mean in everyday general practice.

References

1 General Medical Council. *Good Medical Practice* London: General Medical Council; 2006 (available at: www.gmc-uk.org [accessed June 2007]).

2 www.pmetb.org.uk [accessed June 2007].

3 Bullock A, Burke S, Wall D. Curriculum and assessment in higher specialist training *Medical Teacher* 2004; **26(2)**: 174–7.

2 Understanding the curriculum

The curriculum statements

In order to understand how the curriculum works, and how to use it for learning and teaching, you need to understand how it is constructed. This involves familiarising yourself with the curriculum framework (i.e. its basic anatomy).

Figure 2.1

The anatomy of the RCGP curriculum

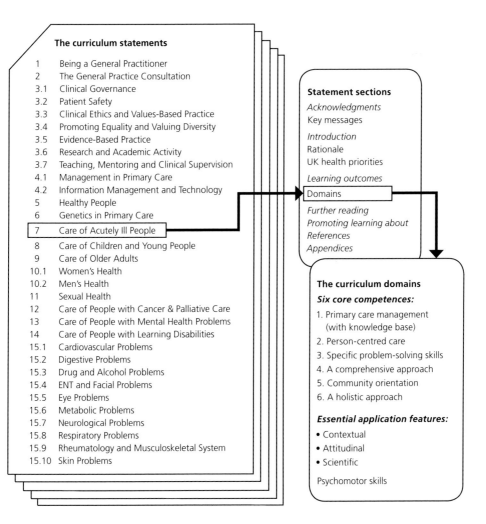

The curriculum statements

1	Being a General Practitioner
2	The General Practice Consultation
3.1	Clinical Governance
3.2	Patient Safety
3.3	Clinical Ethics and Values-Based Practice
3.4	Promoting Equality and Valuing Diversity
3.5	Evidence-Based Practice
3.6	Research and Academic Activity
3.7	Teaching, Mentoring and Clinical Supervision
4.1	Management in Primary Care
4.2	Information Management and Technology
5	Healthy People
6	Genetics in Primary Care
7	Care of Acutely Ill People
8	Care of Children and Young People
9	Care of Older Adults
10.1	Women's Health
10.2	Men's Health
11	Sexual Health
12	Care of People with Cancer & Palliative Care
13	Care of People with Mental Health Problems
14	Care of People with Learning Disabilities
15.1	Cardiovascular Problems
15.2	Digestive Problems
15.3	Drug and Alcohol Problems
15.4	ENT and Facial Problems
15.5	Eye Problems
15.6	Metabolic Problems
15.7	Neurological Problems
15.8	Respiratory Problems
15.9	Rheumatology and Musculoskeletal System
15.10	Skin Problems

Statement sections

Acknowledgments
Key messages
Introduction
Rationale
UK health priorities
Learning outcomes
Domains
Further reading
Promoting learning about
References
Appendices

The curriculum domains

Six core competences:

1. Primary care management
   (with knowledge base)
2. Person-centred care
3. Specific problem-solving skills
4. A comprehensive approach
5. Community orientation
6. A holistic approach

Essential application features:

• Contextual
• Attitudinal
• Scientific

Psychomotor skills

The first thing you will notice when viewing the curriculum is that it is made up of 32 *curriculum statements*. These statements describe the range of professional responsibilities required of a modern GP. The curriculum statements can be freely accessed on the RCGP curriculum website (www.rcgp-curriculum.org.uk). You may find it useful to have access to the curriculum statements while reading this chapter.

Some of the statements describe the professional and managerial aspects of general practice, some describe the care of special groups of people and some describe specific clinical topics. To use an analogy, each statement is like a different breed of dog; each has the same basic features but a slightly different appearance.

The first statement, *Being a General Practitioner*, is the most important. This statement is referred to as the *core statement* of the curriculum, as it outlines what being a GP is all about (see Chapter 6, 'The core competences', for more details). The core statement forms the template on which all the other curriculum statements are based. To continue the dog analogy, the core statement is the common ancestor (the wolf) from which all the other statements (the different breeds of dog) are descended.

How each curriculum statement is constructed

On opening a curriculum statement, you will see that it contains the following content sections:

- An *acknowledegments* section, where the people who helped create the statement are recognised and the *key messages* of the statement are listed.

- An *introduction* section, which includes the *rationale* for why this particular statement has been written and the relevant *UK health priorities* that set the scene, such as National Service Frameworks,[1] national guidelines and other important health policies.

- The *learning outcomes* section describes the knowledge, skills and attitudes that must be mastered to demonstrate competence in this particular topic area. This section is subdivided into the *curriculum domains* and the *knowledge base*.

- A *further reading* section with guidance on some relevant teaching and learning resources, and other useful information.

- A *references* section with indexed references and a bibliography.

- Some statements have additional sections with information on promoting learning and some also contain appendices.

The learning outcomes

The most important educational part of each curriculum statement is its learning outcomes section. Nearly all of the educational content of the curriculum is found here.

As expected, the learning outcomes section contains the learning outcomes for each statement. Each individual *learning outcome* is a brief description of the knowledge, skill, attitude or area of expertise that a GP must master. In some of the curriculum statements, the individual learning outcomes have been put into groups, which together make up an everyday GP task. These everyday tasks are known as *competencies.*[i]

To achieve a competency, a learner must first master the individual learning outcomes and develop the ability to put these together purposefully to perform the task to a professional standard.

Table 2.1

An example of a competency and its associated learning outcomes	
Competency	1.1 To manage primary contact with patients, dealing with unselected problems
Learning outcomes	*This requires*
	1. Knowledge of the epidemiology of problems presenting in primary care
	2. Mastering an approach that allows easy access for patients with unselected problems
	3. An organisational approach to the management of chronic conditions
	4. Knowledge of conditions encountered in primary care and their treatment

The curriculum domains and knowledge base

The curriculum domains

You will note that the learning outcomes section of each statement is arranged into a number of subsections, referred to as the *curriculum domains*. There are 10 domains in the curriculum: six *domains of core competence*, three *essential application features*, and one for *psychomotor skills*.

The curriculum domains form an extremely useful framework

---

i The term *competencies* (as in everyday GP tasks) should be distinguished from the term *competences* (as in the six core competences of general practice).

for learning the fundamentals of general practice – so useful, in fact, that we have devoted a considerable chunk of this book to exploring the domains in detail and explaining how to learn or teach them (see Chapter 6, 'The core competences'). Understanding the curriculum domains is also crucial if you want to understand how the new MRCGP assessments work (see Chapter 5, 'Succeeding at the new MRCGP').

The six domains of core competence

A core competence is a broad area of expertise that is fundamentally important to general practice. The six domains of core competence of general practice are also referred to, in the curriculum, as the '*six core competences*' for short.

The six domains of core competence of general practice[3] are:

1. Primary care management

2. Person-centred care

3. Specific problem-solving skills

4. A comprehensive approach

5. Community orientation

6. A holistic approach.

Each of the six core competences is explored in detail in Chapter 6, 'The core competences'.

Although every topic statement contains the same six domains of core competence, the emphasis given to each domain of competence is greater in some statements than in others. For example, in statement 12, *Cancer and Palliative Care*, the holistic approach domain is particularly apparent, whereas in 7, *Acutely Ill People*, the primary care management domain is more prominent.

The essential application features

Partnering the six domains of core competence are three *essential application features*:

1. **Contextual** – using the context of the person, the family, the community and their culture

2. **Attitudinal** – basing actions on the doctor's professional capabilities, values and ethics

3. **Scientific** – adopting a critical and research-based approach to practice and maintaining this through continuing learning and quality improvement.

Each essential application feature describes a fundamental aspect of general practice that determines how a GP actually performs his or her professional duties. The important word is 'application' – the three essential application features exert a strong influence over how a GP applies his or her acquired knowledge and skills in real-life situations.

For example, a GP may appear to be acting competently by deciding to refer a sick patient to hospital, but this may actually be evidence of incompetence if the GP has failed to take the wishes of the patient into account or to consider using a more appropriate community-based service. This demonstrates the importance of applying skills and knowledge according to the context of the local environment. For this reason, it is essential for a GP to master the application features if he or she is to perform competently in his or her everyday practice.

The three essential application features are explained in more detail in Chapter 6, 'The core competences'.

The core competences and essential application features were published by the European Academy of Teachers in General Practice (EURACT) in their *European Definition of General Practice/Family Medicine*.[2] The competences were originally developed by WONCA,[ii] the World Organization of National Colleges, Academies and Academic Associations of General Practitioners and Family Physicians.

---

ii Not to be confused with Wonka, the amazing chocolatier!

Table 2.2

The curriculum phrase book	
Curriculum statement	One of the 32 documents that together make up the RCGP Curriculum for Specialty Training for General Practice
Learning outcome	A specific piece of knowledge, skill, attitude or area of expertise that a GP should acquire
Competency	An everyday task that a GP must be able to perform to a professional standard (usually requiring mastery of a group of several learning outcomes)
Core competence	One of the six domains of core competence of general practice: primary care management, person-centred care, specific problem-solving skills, a comprehensive approach, community orientation and a holistic approach
Essential application feature	A fundamental aspect of general practice that determines how a GP applies his or her knowledge and skills in a real-life situation: contextual, attitudinal and scientific
Curriculum domain	A generic term for the 10 sections that form the educational framework of the curriculum, including: the six core competences, the three essential application features and the psychomotor skills
Psychomotor skills	The practical and clinical skills a GP must master, such as using an otoscope or taking a cervical smear
The knowledge base	The key items of knowledge included within some of the curriculum statements that a GP is expected to acquire as a basic foundation for general practice
The new MRCGP syllabus	A description of the knowledge, skills, attitudes and other attributes that candidates may be expected to demonstrate to successfully complete the nMRCGP assessments

Psychomotor skills

Some statements contain a section for describing the psychomotor skills that a GP must develop in that particular topic area. Psycho-motor skills are the everyday practical and clinical skills that GPs perform. Examples include basic life support skills, taking a cervical smear, using an ophthalmoscope or doing a clinical examination.

The knowledge base

In addition to the 10 curriculum domains, the curriculum contains a syllabus of core knowledge, referred to as the *knowledge base*. The knowledge base is located within the primary care management domain in a number of the curriculum statements (Chapter 7, 'The essential knowledge', contains the condensed knowledge base for every curriculum statement).

The knowledge base is a list of items of knowledge that a GP is expected to acquire as a basic foundation to general practice. The knowledge items in each statement are organised into the following categories:

- Symptoms

- Common and important conditions

- Investigations

- Treatment

- Emergency care

- Prevention.

The new MRCGP syllabus

A new MRCGP syllabus has also been created as an adjunct to the curriculum. The new MRCGP syllabus provides a summary of the knowledge, skills, attitudes and other attributes that will be tested in the new MRCGP assessments. It is available on the RCGP curriculum website: www.rcgp-curriculum.org.uk.

In educational terms, a syllabus is not the same as a curriculum – a curriculum encompasses all the complex factors that contribute to a comprehensive educational programme; this includes the rationale for learning a topic, the context where learning takes place and the ways in which learning can be achieved. A syllabus, on the other hand, is simply concerned with specifying a list of items that can be learned, taught or assessed.

Similarly, the new MRCGP syllabus is a subpart of the RCGP curriculum, and is concerned with specifying topics that should be assessed by the new MRCGP. This is described in more detail in Chapter 5, 'Succeeding at the new MRCGP'.

As you might expect, the content of the new MRCGP syllabus overlaps considerably with the curriculum knowledge base. Chapter 7 of this book, 'The essential knowledge', includes the items of knowledge and practical skills included in the curriculum knowledge base as well as other topics included in the new MRCGP syllabus. We have also included some handy tips on how to learn or teach these.

Feedback on the curriculum

The RCGP curriculum website has a section where users of the curriculum can ask questions and read advice on using the curriculum in practice. You can also email your feedback on the curriculum and the new MRCGP to the Royal College of General Practitioners at: postgraduatetraining@rcgp.org.uk.

References

1   www.library.nhs.uk [accessed June 2007].

2   WONCA. *The European Definition of General Practice/Family Medicine* Barcelona: World Health Organization, 2002.

3   RCGP curriculum statement 1: *Being a General Practitioner* London: RCGP, 2007.

3 Learning the curriculum

How GPs learn

There are a number of key principles that make learning more effective for adults, which have been identified from many years of research. These principles of adult learning are particularly relevant for GPs – if they are applied successfully in general practice, learning will be more effective:

1 GPs learn from experience

Learning in most adults is generally more effective when it is based on real experience rather than abstract theory alone. For a GP, learning from experience involves reflecting on (i.e. 'thinking about') events that occur in daily practice, considering why these feel significant, addressing any learning needs that arise and formulating a new approach that can be adopted in the future. Then, the next time a similar situation recurs, the GP's response will be different; this leads to another new experience, a further opportunity for reflection, and so on. This reflective learning cycle can repeat *ad infinitum* and each time it occurs something new can be learned. This is the cycle of experiential and reflective learning.[1]

2 GPs like to direct their own learning

Most adults like to feel in charge of their lives and the same applies to their learning, although there are times when we want to be told what learning activities to do rather than find out for ourselves. This is particularly the case when a learner is under stress or adjusting to a new learning environment. Specialty registrars who are just starting out in general practice often request a considerable amount of direction from their trainers and course organisers initially, although they tend to take more and more control of their learning as their experience and confidence grows. This principle is referred to as self-directed learning.[2]

3 GPs learn what they need to learn

For many GPs, their readiness to learn is often strongly related to how relevant they perceive a learning activity to be to the tasks they perform in their day-to-day role. In other words, learning based on the curriculum needs to feel relevant to learning how to be a GP, passing the new MRCGP assessments, or getting through appraisal and revalidation, or many learners will lose interest. This principle is known as needs-based learning.

4 GPs learn how to solve problems

Traditionally, lessons at school are categorised into subjects. In medical school, we call these 'topics' or 'specialties'. Unfortunately for GPs, however, patients in the real world do not often present with their complaints neatly categorised. A competent GP must learn to apply his or her medical expertise effectively to daily situations, based on the underlying theoretical medical knowledge and theory he or she has previously acquired. This is the principle behind problem-based learning.[3]

Learning from experience in general practice

The learning acquired in medical school that is based on theoretical topics is an essential foundation for general practice, but this form of education is traditionally focused on learning *about medicine* rather than learning *how to be a doctor*. This is similar to the difference between learning the mechanics of how a car works and learning how to drive. One of the best ways to learn to be a competent GP is by undertaking learning activities based in real-life situations, addressing the unpredictable problems that arise when seeing real patients. This is the rationale for developing training programmes based on problem-based learning (also referred to as problem-centred learning).

Doctors often gain their first experience of consulting in general practice while sitting in with their trainer and observing other, established GPs and primary-care professionals. These early experiences may be very influential in determining the behaviours that a fledgling GP will adopt in his or her own professional practice. As time progresses, supervised surgeries are gradually replaced by unsupervised surgeries, initially supported with regular 'debriefing' time.

Shared surgeries, preferably arranged with a number of different GPs to provide variety, are extremely helpful at regular intervals throughout the training period (and even beyond) as they expose a GP trainee to a range of alternative consulting styles and techniques. Shared surgeries also provide trainees with the opportunity to gain valuable real-time feedback about their performance from other GPs.[4]

Reflective learning

Reflection is an important stage of the learning process in general practice. This requires learners to successfully develop the skills of reflection *on practice* and reflection *in practice*.[5,6] Reflection *on practice* involves thinking back to a situation in the past, such as a consultation, and recalling what happened and considering the feelings generated at that time by the experience. Both the events and the feelings are analysed and explored to identify any significant learning points (Description → Feelings → Analysis → Conclusion). The purpose of analysing the experience in this way is to transform it from a vague emotional memory into usable knowledge and helpful understanding that can be adopted in future practice.

Figure 3.1

An example of reflection on practice

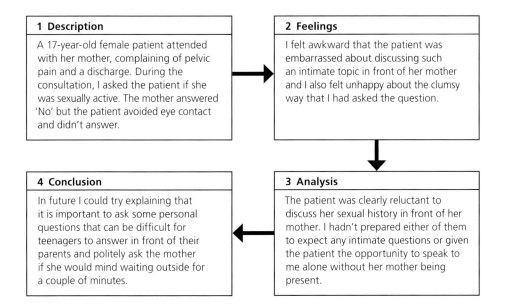

1 Description

A 17-year-old female patient attended with her mother, complaining of pelvic pain and a discharge. During the consultation, I asked the patient if she was sexually active. The mother answered 'No' but the patient avoided eye contact and didn't answer.

2 Feelings

I felt awkward that the patient was embarrassed about discussing such an intimate topic in front of her mother and I also felt unhappy about the clumsy way that I had asked the question.

4 Conclusion

In future I could try explaining that it is important to ask some personal questions that can be difficult for teenagers to answer in front of their parents and politely ask the mother if she would mind waiting outside for a couple of minutes.

3 Analysis

The patient was clearly reluctant to discuss her sexual history in front of her mother. I hadn't prepared either of them to expect any intimate questions or given the patient the opportunity to speak to me alone without her mother being present.

Reflection *in practice* involves reflecting in real time, while a situation is ongoing, and adjusting your behaviour accordingly. For example, a GP with underdeveloped reflective skills may experience feelings of anger during a challenging consultation and respond by growing increasingly angry him or herself, only to regret his or her behaviour afterwards. A GP with highly developed reflective skills would recognise his or her growing feelings of anger and take action to deal with them appropriately, possibly by sharing his or her feelings with the patient; 'I would like to help you but I'm finding it difficult to think of how to do this as I am feeling increasingly frustrated myself ...'

GPs with strong reflective preferences may spend a lot of time ruminating on past events, whereas those with activist tendencies may find reflection more of an uphill struggle. In either case, it is important that reflection should be a constructive process with tangible rather than imaginary benefits. Reflection can be aided by a variety of techniques; natural introverts and reflectors may prefer personal reflective diaries and one-to-one debriefing sessions. Those with more extrovert and activist preferences, however, may prefer to reflect through discussion with their peers, debates in learning groups and direct feedback.[7]

Self-directed learning in general practice

An effective self-directed approach to learning involves far more than spending an hour each week in a tutorial discussing any interesting patients that spring to mind! A self-directed approach actually requires a lot of planning and organisation; tutorials and other educational activities should be planned in advance to create a personalised programme of educational experiences. In other words, each learning activity should be designed to meet specific objectives based on the learner's identified learning needs, and the particular educational activities chosen should be tailored to complement the learner's individual learning preferences.

It is unrealistic, however, to expect new specialty registrars to arrive in general practice with all the learning skills required to adopt a fully self-directed approach to their learning. Most experienced trainers recognise this and arrange an induction programme involving a number of prearranged educational activities for the first few weeks, encouraging their trainees to take on more responsibility for managing their own learning as their self-directed learning skills develop. More information on arranging an induction programme for specialty registrars can be found in Chapter 4, 'Teaching the curriculum'.

The ability to create a personal development plan (PDP) is an important aspect of self-directed professional learning and this key skill is increasingly important for GPs undergoing annual appraisal and revalidation. More tips and advice on this are included below.

Learning what you need to learn

One of the first questions every new GP trainee asks is 'What do I need to learn to be a GP?' Although many answers to this question exist, very few of these are particularly helpful to the learner.

- 'Learn a bit about everything ...'
- 'Only you can decide what you need to learn ...'
- 'Learn the RCGP curriculum ...'

General practice is a very broad specialty and the curriculum is similarly broad – the first step every GP in training must do when planning his or her learning is to identify his or her learning needs in order to set some priorities.

GP learners can identify their individual learning needs through a large number of educational activities. Some of these are listed in Table 3.1.

Table 3.1

Popular activities for identifying learning needs in general practice

1 Activities performed by the learner
- Reflective practice
- ○ Keeping a reflective diary of consultations
- ○ Keeping a log of referrals and investigations
- ○ Reflection on learning experiences
- ○ Reflection on an issue at intervals over time

- Self-assessment of knowledge and skills
- ○ Completing a confidence rating scale (e.g. Chapter 7, 'The essential knowledge')
- ○ Reviewing the outcomes of referrals
- ○ Reviewing a targeted or random selection of case notes

- Self-directed learning activities
- ○ Reading journal articles and textbooks
- ○ Completing e-learning modules
- ○ Viewing the internet/TV/media

2 Activities performed with others
- Learning needs identified with patients
- ○ Recording difficulties arising in day-to-day practice
- ○ Asking for informal feedback from patients
- ○ Getting patients to complete satisfaction questionnaires
- ○ Video analysis of consultations

Continued over

- Learning needs identified by educational activities
- ○ Recording learning needs arising out of tutorials
- ○ Identifying learning needs in shared surgeries
- ○ Learning needs identified by problem-based learning
- ○ Formative assessment and feedback

- Learning needs identified with peers
- ○ Creating presentations for peers
- ○ Organising and leading group teaching activities
- ○ Attending courses and educational meetings

- Learning needs identified with the practice team
- ○ Discussing issues arising in practice meetings
- ○ Obtaining 360° feedback from the practice team
- ○ Undertaking a Significant Event Analysis

3 Activities that use the RCGP curriculum
- Learner self-assessment
- ○ Assessing your own competency against the core competences
- ○ Testing your own knowledge against the knowledge base
- ○ Judging your own behaviour against the curriculum outcomes

- Formative assessment
- ○ Undertaking Workplace-Based Assessment (WPBA)

- Using the curriculum domains grid (see Appendix 1).

Source: www.trainingpractice.co.uk.

Chapter 7 of this guide, 'The essential knowledge', has also been designed as a confidence rating scale (an electronic version of this is available from www.rcgp-curriculum.org.uk). This allows learners to score themselves on their 'level of confidence' for a list of topics from the curriculum. This can be a useful way for a new specialty registrar to start prioritising his or her learning needs, although it is important to remember that a confidence score may not always accurately reflect a true level of ability!

Another useful tool for prioritising learning needs is RCGP Scotland's PEP eKit – an online interactive test of general practice.[i] Contact with patients will generate many learning needs on a daily basis, particularly at the start of training, which can be recorded in a patient log or learning portfolio. More complex learning needs can be identified by case analysis, consultation analysis (video surgeries) and shared surgeries.

These methods and other ways of identifying learning needs are explained in more detail in Chapter 4, 'Teaching the curricu-

[i] Available from RCGP Scotland. Go to www.pep-ekit.org.uk or email pep-ekit@rcgp-scotland.org.uk.

lum', along with some tools for identifying individual learning styles and preferences.

Problem-based learning in primary care

Many of the learning needs that arise in daily practice are relatively simple (e.g. a need to find out a simple piece of factual knowledge) and can be simply recorded in a logbook or spreadsheet and dealt with on a daily basis.

With the advent of rapid internet access, a number of web-based resources now exist that can enable GPs to address simple learning needs during the consultation, meaning that learning occurs immediately and feels highly relevant.

Table 3.2

An example of a simple learning need arising during a consultation	
Problem	An 18-year-old student attends with abdominal bloating and intermittent loose stools
Comments	History suggests irritable bowel syndrome, but I decide I ought to exclude coeliac disease – only I can't remember which is the best blood investigation for this …?
Learning need	Learn the best blood test for excluding coeliac disease
Action taken	Looked up on www.gpnotebook.co.uk during the consultation. Best screening test is anti-endomyseal antibody test, which has a sensitivity of over 95% in the presence of normal IgA
Outcome	Blood test taken – antibody result is negative with normal IgA, effectively ruling out coeliac disease in this context. Patient is started on anti-spasmodic treatment for IBS; symptoms much better at review two weeks later!

Problem-based case analysis

Complex cases can form the basis of problem-based discussions in tutorials and group learning. Cases can be selected by random (incorporating the element of surprise) or from a logbook recording the most challenging cases encountered.

Tutorials

Tutorials based on particular topics (e.g. gut problems) have a role when a specific learning need in this area has been identified, and are often most effective when both the trainee and the trainer have had the opportunity to prepare in advance. Once the theoretical knowledge has been covered, it is often very useful to discuss how the knowledge can be applied to real-life cases, as the application of knowledge requires a higher level of learning and it is at this stage when the difficulties often emerge.

Learning complex skills

Learning needs arising from problem-based cases that involve the development of complex GP skills, attitudes or expertise require a more sophisticated approach. This includes communication skills, consultation techniques and dealing with ethical dilemmas.

It is often useful to translate these more complex learning needs into personal learning outcomes. A learning outcome is a brief description of a behaviour or activity that the learner is able to demonstrate, the context where it will be demonstrated, the standard to which it will be performed, and the timescale in which it will be achieved.

Table 3.3

An example of a personal learning outcome

The activity	I will be able to negotiate shared management plans with patients …
The context	… in my everyday consultations …
The standard	… to the standard required to practise independently as a GP …
The timescale	… by the completion of my GP training

As with curriculum learning outcomes, personal learning outcomes can be further broken down into their component parts – knowledge, attitudes and skills – and these component parts can be addressed as part of a personal learning plan (PLP) involving a range of different learning activities.

Learning in groups

The half-day release courses run by vocational training programmes are generally very popular among specialty registrars.[ii] This is partly because learning groups provide important functions that extend far beyond the simple educational aims of the particular group activity. For example, many specialty registrars

ii Well anything's better than real work, right?!

particularly value the opportunity to meet with fellow trainees in order to share experiences with patients ('horror stories') and chat about how they are tackling their learning. Being a specialty registrar can feel quite isolated at times, especially as few practices are able to take more than one new learner at a time; a weekly meeting with a group of peers performs an important 'housekeeping' function for many trainees.[8]

In order to deliver GP education in line with PMETB requirements, training programme directors are offering specialty registrars more say in the planning of their group learning programmes. This is also important to ensure that learning in groups is self-directed and needs based, otherwise the educational activities of the group may become increasingly irrelevant to individual learners.

Research suggests that learning groups are most productive if they are facilitated effectively, although many groups can eventually become productive by themselves if given sufficient time to develop.[9] Many specialty registrars, trainers and newly qualified GPs form their own informal learning groups to help them prepare for assessments or to facilitate continuing professional development.

Group learning can be particularly useful for the shaping of attitudes and also act as professional 'barometers' against which individual GPs may judge their own professional opinions and values. Groups are the perfect setting to debate wider ethical and professional issues, often arising from difficult cases, the learning of which requires the consideration of points of view that are necessarily different from one's own.

Learning from other health professionals

An essential part of being a doctor involves teaching and learning from other health professionals. This is increasingly the case in general practice. A GP may be involved, either directly or indirectly, in educational activities with medical students, Foundation-year doctors, specialty registrars, established GPs and other healthcare professionals and staff members in the practice.

Spending time with other primary healthcare team workers and other related professionals (such as community pharmacists and physios) is often very useful.

Table 3.4

Learning from other healthcare professionals	
Spend time with	**Particularly good for learning**
Practice nurses	Chronic disease management, routine vaccinations and travel immunisations, dressings and wound care, issues that arise when implementing practice protocols or national guidelines, minor illness
District nurses	How to manage chronic disease in the community, dressings and wound care, ulcers, catheterisation and incontinence, local community services, palliative care
Health visitors	Management of common childhood problems such as behavioural difficulties, feeding and toileting, supporting new parents, child protection, vulnerable adults
Community pharmacists	Common prescribing problems, how medications are dispensed, dosette boxes, compliance and concordance
Physiotherapists	How to manage common musculoskeletal complaints, triaging back problems, self-management of back pain

Planning learning activities with the curriculum

The curriculum statements and the curriculum domains (the core competences and essential application features) form a useful framework for planning learning activities. This ensures learning experiences cover all the competency areas of general practice comprehensively. An example using the domains to plan learning activities on cancer and palliative care is included in Table 3.5.

Appendix 1 contains a blank domains matrix grid, which you can photocopy and use as a template to complete your own learning plans. An electronic version is also available at www.rcgp-curriculum.org.uk.

Table 3.5

Using the curriculum domains to plan learning

Example learning activities relating to statement 12:
Care of People with Cancer & Palliative Care

	Essential application features		
Core competences	**Contextual**	**Attitudinal**	**Scientific**
1 **Primary care** **management**	Read the Gold Standards Framework for Palliative Care documents	Discussion with trainer on how my personal experience affects my management	Read textbook section on how to prescribe opioids and other palliative medications
2 **Person-centred** **approach**	Find out how to inform the out-of-hours service about a palliative patient	Read up on the issues around Advanced Directives and capacity to consent	Tutorial arranged on models for the doctor–patient relationship
3 **Specific** **problem-** **solving skills**	Arrange role-plays with actors or colleagues on day release to practise breaking bad news	Discussion planned in Learning Group on the ethics around end-of-life and euthanasia	Go over how to set up a syringe driver with the district nurse
4 **A comprehensive** **approach**	Read up on benefits available for the terminally ill (and the DS1500 form)	Journal club discussion on qualitative research into patients' views on loss of dignity and dying	Review textbook section on the causes of reduced pain threshold (e.g. anxiety, constipation)
5 **Community** **orientation**	Arrange a day with the Macmillan nurse, visiting patients dying at home	Reflect on the NHS end-of-life care document, *Dying at Home*	Identify local risk factors for cancer and prevalence from practice QoF data
6 **A holistic** **approach**	Organise a case-based discussion with trainer on the needs of carers in the practice	Ask colleagues how they would ask a palliative patient about spiritual care needs	Read up on the key models of bereavement and important sources of support

Learning in secondary care

Many acute medical and surgical jobs provide great experience of managing seriously ill patients in hospital. In the UK, however, a GP does not usually spend very long managing a patient who is obviously seriously ill, beyond administering immediate emergency care until an ambulance arrives, or caring for a terminally ill patient at home. A hospital job, therefore, can be a great opportunity to learn how to examine, investigate and manage patients with serious illnesses and for practising specific psychomotor skills (like joint injections or taking a smear).

Table 3.6

Useful learning opportunities in secondary care	
Spend time in	**Particularly good for learning**
Outpatient clinics	Secondary-care management, consulting with patients, how specialists manage specialised conditions, familiarity with serious illness, developing specific clinical and psychomotor skills
Consultant ward-rounds	Bedside teaching and getting consultant feedback on clinical and decision-making skills
Multidisciplinary team meetings	How multidisciplinary teams work together and communicate
Educational meetings	A range of specialist educational topics

GPs must learn how to distinguish patients who may be *seriously ill* and need to go to hospital from the far larger group of patients presenting in the community with symptoms but without serious illness, the vast majority of whom never trouble secondary care. Most secondary-care jobs, therefore, offer relatively poor opportunities for GPs to learn how to examine, investigate and manage symptomatic patients who do not have serious illnesses, and these skills are best honed during the time spent in general practice.

Learning by teaching

Teaching can be an excellent way to learn – you never fully appreciate what you don't understand until you try to teach it to someone else! The need for GPs to develop teaching skills is reflected in the curriculum (statement 3.7: *Teaching, Mentoring and Clinical Supervision*). Many specialty registrars taking part in half-day release courses are involved in organising seminars and presentations for their peers as part of their learning programme.

Keeping a learning portfolio

Portfolios are becoming increasingly popular in ongoing professional education. A professional development or learning portfolio is a collection of evidence that enables a GP to record, and reflect on, significant professional events and educational activities. Reflection is an important part of portfolio-based learning, which involves the following steps:

- Identifying your learning needs
- Creating a personal learning plan (PLP) based on these needs
- Using appropriate resources to meet these needs
- Demonstrating what you have learned
- Reflecting on the learning process and identifying new needs.

Table 3.7

A basic PLP template	
Learning need	To successfully manage the concerns of the mother of a child with glue ear and avoid an unnecessary referral
How this was identified	My referrals log and a letter from a local consultant indicate I am referring inappropriately to ENT
Educational activities	1. Read up on the natural history and management of glue ear in an ENT textbook 2. Tutorial planned on eliciting and addressing parental concerns with my trainer 3. Day at the local ENT clinic arranged
Timescale	Six weeks
Evidence of Learning	1. My log shows I successfully reduced my referrals 2. Scored 87% in an ENT e-learning module 3. Positive feedback from trainer on video consultations

Portfolio learning is becoming integrated into medical training. Foundation doctors are required to keep a portfolio as part of their training and GP specialty registrars use the RCGP's web-based electronic portfolio to complete their Workplace-Based Assessment as part of the new MRCGP assessment. This forms an excellent base for a newly qualified GP to continue building a personal learning portfolio for the rest of his or her professional career.

Keeping up to date

As medical professionals, GPs are required (and are usually well motivated) to keep their knowledge and skills up to date and develop new skills as they are needed. This process is known as continuing professional development (CPD) and is an essential competency of modern general practice.

Some popular ways of keeping up to date are described in Table 3.8.

Table 3.8

Some popular ways of keeping up to date	
Review the journals	The *British Medical Journal* (BMJ) and the *British Journal of General Practice* (BJGP) contain news and articles of interest to GPs. The journal *Evidence-Based Medicine* contains evidence-based research reviews relevant to primary care. These journals can be accessed online by RCGP members and Associates-in-Training free of charge at www.rcgp.org.uk
Read the GP press	The weekly GP papers include a lot of clinical information and produce a lot of free additional publications that contain information on recent developments in primary care
Journal watch	Several organisations, including the RCGP, offer an electronic journal watch service, which highlights and summarises the latest relevant research findings
Hot topics	A number of courses offer GPs 'refreshers' on current topics of importance in general practice
NICE guidelines	You can get on the NICE mailing list and receive its regular updates and new guidelines free of charge (www.nice.org.uk)

CPD has been defined as 'lifelong learning for all individuals and teams, enabling professionals to fulfil their potential while meeting the needs of patients and delivering the health outcomes and health-care priorities of the NHS'.[10]

For a GP, this process involves taking time regularly to identify:

- Personal learning needs

- Practice development needs

- Community and local health service needs.

GPs are required to provide evidence of their ongoing education, create learning plans and demonstrate how they are maintaining and improving their knowledge and skills during their annual appraisal. Once a year, every GP (including GPs in training) must meet with a trained appraiser to review his or her previous year's

PDP and to agree new learning objectives for the following year. The underlying principle of appraisal is that professional development should be driven by individual needs and priorities.

The online NHS appraisals toolkit (www.appraisals.nhs.uk) is a popular tool among GPs. It offers guidance on appraisal and practical tools for recording evidence of learning and personal development learning plans, as well as offering access to online advice from peers and experienced appraisers.

References

1 Kolb DA. *Experiential Learning: experience as the source of learning and development* New Jersey: Prentice Hall, 1984.

2 Brookfield S D. *Understanding and Facilitating Adult Learning* San Francisco: Jossey-Bass, 1986.

3 Knowles M S. *Andragogy in Action: applying modern principles of adult learning* San Francisco: Jossey-Bass, 1984.

4 Middleton P and Field S J. *The GP Trainer's Handbook* Oxford: Radcliffe Medical Press, 2001.

5 Schön D. *The Reflective Practitioner* New York: Basic Books, 1983.

6 Schön D. *Educating the Reflective Practitioner* San Francisco: Jossey-Bass, 1987.

7 Honey P and Mumford A. *Manual of Learning Styles* London: P. Honey, 1982.

8 As per Neighbour's five-checkpoint consultation model. Neighbour R. *The Inner Consultation* Lancaster: MTP, 1987.

9 Tuckman B and Jensen M. Stages of small group development *Group and Organizational Studies* 1977; **2**: 419–27.

10 NHS Executive. *Continuing Professional Development: quality in the new NHS* Leeds: NHS Executive, 1999.

4 Teaching the curriculum

Modern GP training

Since the first vocational training schemes were established in the 1960s, general practice training has become progressively more trainee-centred. In the future, emphasis will increasingly fall on active learning rather than on the passive acquisition of knowledge. It will also focus on the assessment of clinical competences rather than on the ability to retain and recall facts.

The well-established approach of regular protected time outside the practice, typically through a weekly half-day release programme, has been praised over the years and was assessed positively in a national survey of GP educators and trainees in 2006.[1] Despite the success of their half-day release courses, however, training programmes will need to be flexible and adaptable to change; feedback from trainees and patient participation should feed into the construction of learning programmes throughout the three-year specialty training programme for general practice.

The RCGP curriculum reflects these developments in education, as well as the changing role of medicine in society and the growing expectations patients have of their GP. This chapter provides practical advice on teaching general practice and offers guidance for trainers and other GP educators who are involved in supporting the trainees' learning of the curriculum on a day-to-day basis.

The role of the GP trainer

The GP trainer forms the bedrock of general practice training in the UK. The role is challenging and diverse; it encompasses the responsibilities of critical friend, supervisor, educator, assessor, mentor, pastoral carer and role model. These roles are complex and may, at times, come into conflict. Furthermore, the new three-year specialty training programme brings additional responsibilities for trainers throughout the entire three-year programme, including the placements in secondary care, in addition to the responsibilities during the general practice placement.

The relationship between the specialty registrar and his or her trainer is at the heart of the teaching and learning process, whereby trainees acquire and develop the knowledge, skills and attitudes needed to become an effective GP. It is the primary responsibility of the trainer to oversee and support the specialty registrar's educational progress. To do this, a trainer must have the appropriate professional attributes, personal qualities and training required for the task.

Specialty registrars will derive most of their useful learning from seeing and contributing to good-quality patient care. One of the greatest influences on them is the example given by their trainer as a doctor – their role model. For this reason, a GP trainer must be an enthusiastic, competent, communicative and caring GP, working in a well-organised practice.[i] He or she must also be expected to know and accept the responsibilities of his or her role.

A trainer's enthusiasm for general practice must also apply to his or her own personal learning and willingness to develop further as a clinical teacher. Trainers require additional knowledge and skills over and above those of their non-teaching colleagues and their contribution to learning activities outside the practice is often a good illustration of a wider commitment to education. Trainers must devote time to prepare carefully for their training responsibilities and may benefit from wider teaching experience, for example with medical students or other health professionals. They should be willing to be appraised by their peers as this encourages their trainees to adopt a similar critical approach to their work.

Creating a good training environment

The effectiveness of learning is greatly influenced by the environment in which the learning occurs.[2] For specialty registrars to get the most out of their training experiences in general practice, their training practice must offer a high standard of care and be run efficiently. GP specialty registrars learn a lot from seeing how the principles of clinical governance and high professional standards are put into daily practice.

---

i The ability to leap over tall buildings is optional!

Table 4.1

Features of a good training environment	
Patients	To gain a wide enough range of experience to cover the core domains of competence, specialty registrars need a good mix of patients. They also need to be supported when dealing with difficult or demanding patients
GPs and other practitioners	Specialty registrars should be exposed to a range of consulting styles and encouraged to spend time with all the various members of the primary healthcare team (see Chapter 3, 'Learning the curriculum')
Premises	Specialty registrars need their own private space for reflective learning, reading and educational work. They obviously need a consulting room too!
Equipment	As well as clinical equipment, specialty registrars need access to a video camera, a TV and DVD/video player to aid in the development of consultation skills, and a projector/laptop for presentations and seminars
Educational resources	All training practices should have a library stocked with relevant books (like this one!) although many learning resources are now electronic or web-based. Specialty registrars must have access to an NHS internet-linked computer and be able to rapidly access educational resources such as the RCGP curriculum website: www.rcgp-curriculum.org.uk
Teamwork and management	Specialty registrars need to learn how effective teams work. They should feel involved in practice meetings and be encouraged to become involved in projects with other team members. Training practices need clear management systems in place, including those for appointments, phone messages, repeat prescribing, home visit requests, referrals, staff communication and team leadership
Audit and quality assurance	An attitude of striving for continual improvement is extremely important in a learning organisation. Ongoing monitoring by the practice of its standard of care and a willingness to make changes is a fundamental part of good practice

Preparing to teach the curriculum

As part of the submission to the Postgraduate Medical Education and Training Board (PMETB), the RCGP proposed a new model of learning for general practice that combined three important aspects:

- The importance of balance and diversity in the learning situations that trainees experience

- An emphasis on clarity and transparency of learning outcomes as professional, adult learners expect
- Recognition of the distinctive requirements of GPs as adult learners.

The GP trainer, as guide and mentor, has a central role in supporting his or her specialty registrar through the training and, by working closely with local programme directors and deanery staff, will ensure that these three elements are addressed throughout the length of the three-year training programme.

Balance and diversity

Learning and teaching take place in a variety of educational environments, including hospital settings and the GP practice. In addition to training in the workplace, the GP trainee takes part in the formal learning opportunities provided through departmental teaching sessions, seminars and day-release group activities. Learning and teaching in all these contexts will be aided by clarity of the expected outcomes, which are specified in terms of the learning outcomes described in the curriculum.

The domains of competence

The six domains of core competence[ii] define the steps on the way to expertise, specifically the ability to use knowledge, understanding, thinking and practical skills to perform to the national standards required in employment. A GP who is competent has general attributes incorporating understanding and judgement: 'a complex structuring of attributes needed for intelligent performance in specific situations'.[3] The domains of competence are simultaneously building blocks of professional competence and inter-related parts of an integrated – holistic – whole.

Teaching based on adult learning principles

The teaching and learning of general practice should be organised with attention to the principles of adult learning: learning should be self-directed, experiential, needs-based and problem-centred. A summary of these key principles is set out in Chapter 3, 'Learning the curriculum'.

---

ii See Chapter 2, 'Understanding the curriculum', for a full explanation of the core competences.
iii Lave and Wenger (1991) define apprenticeship as the development of professional expertise through 'legitimate peripheral participation in a community of practice'.

The apprenticeship model

The primary relationship in GP training exists between the trainer (the educator) and the trainee (the learner). This relationship is embedded in daily professional working practice; apprenticeship blends daily professional work with education to enable the development of expertise.[iii,4]

The medical profession has adopted apprenticeship as its main model of training since before the time of Hippocrates. A key strength of apprenticeship as a model for GP training is the opportunity it offers a trainee to develop genuinely useful and relevant skills, and also to assimilate professional values from more experienced colleagues. A great deal of 'hidden learning' takes place subconsciously through the observation of experienced GPs at work. Such learning is subtle and hard to quantify; learners may not be aware of what they have learned until they move to a situation where they see things done less proficiently.

The apprenticeship model also sits well with the principles of adult learning, especially if provision is made for reflection with the use of personal reflective diaries and case-based discussions. Because of the need to provide a first response to any patient who may present, general practice involves a different balance of skills and knowledge from other branches of medicine. The key is experience combined with reflection; learners must be exposed to a high number of contacts with patients to hone their skills.

The informal curriculum

While the RCGP has invested considerable energy into developing an official curriculum for GP training, the 'informal curriculum' is also an important component of a specialty registrar's learning. The informal curriculum is the term used to describe what trainees learn from a variety of sources and interactions while taking part in extracurricular activities.[5] The trainer has a role in ensuring that there is sufficient flexibility and time for the specialty registrar to make the most of educational opportunities available outside of work and the formal teaching programme.

The hidden curriculum

The 'hidden curriculum' is what the specialty registrar learns but the trainer did not set out to teach! Every learner's interactions with his or her trainer, peers, faculty, and others in the hospital or general practice setting will have an impact on his or her development as a GP, his or her qualities and values, and how he or she interacts with others.

The degree of professionalism exhibited by role models can exert an important influence on a learner's professional development. The trainer should be aware that this will have already occurred from previous experiences and he or she may encounter a specialty registrar who encountered poor role models during his or her education or early medical training. Many have had personal experience of teachers who intimidate and humiliate their students, which discourages participation and has a negative effect on learning.

All doctors should be aware that the way trainees are treated may influence the way the trainee, in turn, will learn to behave. A doctor may not consider this when making a demeaning remark about a patient, a patient's relative, a nurse, or a colleague, even if it is not meant seriously. We need to create an environment in the practice where the 'hidden curriculum' reinforces, rather than undermines, our professional ideals.

Induction of a new specialty registrar

Induction is an important process to lay the foundation for learning in all organisations. The General Medical Council (GMC) and PMETB both believe that induction is an essential component of an education and training programme. PMETB has developed criteria for approving training posts and programmes that include a section on induction (see Table 4.2).

Table 4.2

Criteria for an induction programme

All programmes must provide induction when a trainee is entering the specialist programme and at the transition from one post to another within a specialist programme. Protected time must be given for induction at each stage. Induction must ensure entrants are informed about:

- The institution and department
- The curriculum
- Assessment and expected learning outcomes from each post within a programme
- Educational and support facilities, and access to them
- Their responsibilities and those of particular members of their local faculty
- How to raise issues of concern, formally and informally
- The basic technical skills needed from day one.

PMETB website: www.pmetb.org.uk.

iv Sometimes called Primary Care Medical Educators (PCMEs).

Many deaneries provide an introduction for all of their specialty registrars to the RCGP curriculum by inviting them to a deanery induction day. Local course organisers[iv] and GP trainers provide the induction for local training programmes, often organised as a staged process over the first few weeks.

Organising an induction programme

The trainer's role in the three-year training programme begins with the induction, and it is therefore a crucial time to start building the educational relationship with the trainee. The style and content of the induction programme will, of course, vary depending on the placement, but a good induction programme usually contains the following elements:

- **Institutional orientation** – details of the NHS's history, culture and values (including information about the training programme plus the placements, in hospital and the training practice)

- **Occupational orientation** – expectations of the role including the terms and conditions of service and health and safety information – this is a legal requirement

- **Organisational orientation** – describing how the specialty registrar fits into the team

- **Physical orientation** – describing the physical environment, buildings, facilities in the placement and programme as a whole

- **Educational orientation** – in detail about the specific placement including an overview of the programme as a whole.

Each trainer will also design an induction programme to fit his or her training practice.[6] This generally runs for the first two to four weeks, depending on individual circumstances. There are often many administrative tasks that require protected time during the induction period, including establishing the registrar's competence on the practice computer system (see condensed statement 4.2: *Information Management and Technology*, in Chapter 7, 'The essential knowledge') and other mundane tasks such as adding his of her details to the practice payroll.

Many training practices provide an introductory booklet or staff handbook, which will build into a useful reference tool for the specialty registrar. This may also be provided in an electronic format. It should contain the agreed induction programme timetable and lots of useful information about the practice, local hospitals and services such as contact details, protocols and guidelines, and, if applicable, a practice formulary.

During the first two weeks it is essential that the specialty registrar is allocated time to get to know a large proportion of the primary healthcare team. This includes other doctors working in the practice, the practice nurses and district nurses, health visitors and midwives, the practice manager and administrative staff, and the receptionists. After the initial induction period, trainees should also spend time with members of the extended primary care team, which will vary depending on the practice and could include chiropodists, community psychiatric nurses, pharmacists, social workers, physiotherapists, optometrists and members of the palliative care team (see Chapter 3, 'Learning the curriculum').

The first two weeks should usually see the specialty registrar progress from sitting in observing the trainer through to conducting consultations with the trainer observing them, to eventually 'flying solo' with long appointment times and the trainer within easy reach. Close supervision is advised during the induction period – it is important to remember that doctors may experience a significant culture shock when they begin in general practice after working in hospital medicine; the trainer or another doctor must always be available for advice or to see a patient if requested.

Table 4.3

The first two weeks – an example induction programme

Week 1

Monday	a.m.	Surgery with GP trainer then home visits with GP trainer
	p.m.	Induction tutorial with GP trainer then surgery with GP trainer
Tuesday	a.m.	Sit in waiting room and observe from patient's perspective then home visits with GP trainer
	p.m.	Induction meeting and tour of practice with practice manager and administrative staff
Wednesday	a.m.	Observe and act as practice receptionist then home visits with GP trainer
	p.m.	Surgery with GP trainer
Thursday	a.m.	Surgery with partner 2
	p.m.	Attend release course (if half-day; this may be an all-day event, which will mean adjusting the timetable)
Friday	a.m.	Surgery with GP trainer then home visits with GP trainer
	p.m.	Practice meeting then tutorial with GP trainer and orientation to RCGP curriculum

Week 2

Monday	a.m.	Surgery with GP trainer then home visits with GP trainer
	p.m.	Tutorial with GP trainer – educational needs assessment
Tuesday	a.m.	Sit in with practice nurse
	p.m.	Surgery with partner 3
Wednesday	a.m.	Surgery on own with space after each case to discuss with GP trainer, then home visits with GP trainer
	p.m.	Baby clinic, meet with health visitor and midwife
Thursday	a.m.	Meet with district nurses and attend their home visits
	p.m.	Attend release course (if half-day; this may be an all-day event, which will mean adjusting the timetable)
Friday	a.m.	Videotaped surgery
	p.m.	Practice meeting followed by tutorial with GP trainer to review videoed consultations

Assessing the learning needs of a new specialty registrar

It is important for the trainer to sit down with the specialty registrar early on in the induction period to discuss learning, so together they can begin to organise a plan to identify and address initial learning needs. It is useful to begin with a review of the specialty registrar's past experience and the knowledge and skills that he or she has acquired so far. There are many aids for the trainer to use at the beginning of training to help identify learning needs and many of these can be used at intervals throughout the training programme.

Self-rating confidence scales

Chapter 7 of this book, 'The essential knowledge', can be used as a confidence rating scale.[v] This enables specialty registrars (and other GPs) to score themselves on their 'level of confidence' for a list of topics covering the breadth of the curriculum. Other examples of confidence rating scales include the Wolverhampton Grid and Manchester Rating Scale.[7] The scales are useful at the beginning of the training programme or an individual placement to help prioritise learning but are not 'outcome measures' and may reflect confidence that is not underpinned by knowledge – the problem of not knowing what you don't know!

v An electronic version is available at www.rcgp-curriculum.org.uk.

PEP eKit

RCGP Scotland has produced the PEP eKit.[vi] This is an online interactive test to help specialty registrars identify strengths, weaknesses and specific educational needs. It is a user-friendly learning tool that can be accessed online anywhere and at any time. It also has a peer review facility that has an option to compare the individual's scores with those of other GPs. It consists of a collection of multiple-choice questions on a range of subjects. The topics covered are ophthalmology, ENT, dermatology, general medicine, psychiatry, paediatrics, obstetrics and gynaecology.

Learning needs identified by patient contact

As specialty registrars conduct more surgeries and have contact with the many patients that they will see each day, they will generate many more identifiable learning needs. They need to capture the moment by recording them in their log or learning portfolio.

PUNs & DENs is a simple system to aid reflective experiential learning, developed in Taunton by Dr Richard Eve.[8] After each consultation, trainees are encouraged to record any patient needs that they felt they had not managed well (PUNS – Patient Unmet Needs); some of these PUNS are the direct result of the doctor's lack of knowledge or skill (DENS – Doctor's Educational Needs). The trainer can use this method to help the specialty registrar reflect on why the patient's needs went unmet and develop an action plan to address the identified learning needs.

Case analysis is an essential weapon in the trainer's armoury. It is a useful tool during a trainee's induction period to identify initial learning needs and may form the basis of many tutorials throughout the three-year training programme. There are a number of types of case analysis:

- Problem case analysis – this involves the selection by the trainer or trainee of cases that are interesting, challenging or problematic. Analysing the cases provides an opportunity to discuss the learning needs that arose and how to deal with them.

- Random case analysis – this is potentially less comfortable and involves randomly selecting cases from surgeries; this enables the trainer to ascertain how the specialty registrar is managing his or her cases and ensure that an appropriate mix of cases is being experienced.

- Analysis of prescriptions, referrals and critical events –

---

vi Available from RCGP Scotland. Go to www.pep-ekit.org.uk or email pep-ekit@rcgp-scotland.org.uk.

these methods provide a wealth of information on the current knowledge and patient management skills of the developing GP.

Consultation analysis

The development of good consulting skills is a key objective of GP training and it is therefore crucial that every specialty registrar's consultations are observed and analysed on a regular basis (see Chapter 7, 'The essential knowledge', on statement 2: *The General Practice Consultation*). This can be done by direct observation by the trainer sitting in with the specialty registrar or by videoing the surgery and playing it back later.

Video consultations formed a major component of the old summative assessment system and, through the new MRCGP consultation observation tool (COT),[vii] it remains an important part of teaching the new curriculum. Videoing of consultations should begin as soon as possible after GP training has commenced, as it is a superb method of identifying learning needs.

Shared surgeries

Regular opportunities for specialty registrars to sit in and observe their trainer and other experienced GPs are part of a well-rounded training experience. Holding shared surgeries with a variety of practitioners enables registrars to:

- Gain feedback on their consultation performance
- See new techniques and approaches being used
- Take advantage of opportunities for case-based discussion
- Arrange to review any patients causing them particular difficulty or concern with an experienced colleague.

Self-awareness assessments

There are a number of techniques available to aid trainers and trainees gain a deeper understanding of their personality, educational preferences and approaches to learning. Most have been developed by educational or organisational psychologists and are questionnaire-based tools, usually available on a commercial basis. They include those concentrating on personality styles, e.g. Myers–Briggs, and learning styles, e.g. Honey and Mumford.

The *Honey and Mumford's Learning Styles Questionnaire*[9] can be a useful tool to help a learner understand his or her learning style

vii See Chapter 5, 'Succeeding at the new MRCGP', for more information on the consultation observation tool and other formative assessment tools.

preferences. Many trainers encourage their trainees to undertake the assessment as part of the induction programme to help plan their subsequent learning activities. The questionnaire is available online and takes about 10–20 minutes. At the end of the session the learner receives an immediate diagnosis of his or her current learning style preferences as well as information about the types of learning activities in keeping with these.

Honey and Mumford assert that it is the learning styles preferences that determine the things people learn from an activity and the ease with which they learn them. They believe that these preferences exert a hidden, but powerful, influence on learning effectiveness. They suggest that if you understand your preferred style, you can apply this understanding to learning new things, and that if you are able to use your natural style, you are likely to find learning easier and quicker. Honey and Mumford divide learners into four distinct types:

Activists enjoy 'doing things' and tend to act first and consider the implications afterwards. They tend to learn best through experience and when dealing with new problems. They need a wide range of activities to keep them engaged and they need to be able to bounce ideas off others. They enjoy chairing meetings, leading discussions and role-playing. They may learn less than others when listening to lectures or from reading, writing or thinking on their own, or when they have to absorb and analyse data.

Theorists like sufficient time to explore and think through problems in a step-by-step manner. They tend to be perfectionists who seek to fit things into a rational scheme. They may appear rather detached and have a tendency to be analytical and objective about ideas. They may learn best when they are given a complex problem where they have to use their skills and knowledge. They want to have the chance to question and investigate ideas behind things. They may find learning difficult when the learning activity is unstructured or when they have to participate in situations that emphasise emotion and feelings.

Pragmatists like opportunities to experiment and tend to be keen to try out what they've learned so they can evaluate its practical use. They prefer to deal with concepts and ideas that can be applied to their role. Pragmatists learn less well when there is no obvious or immediate benefit that they can recognise and prefer to get straight to the point in learning activities, becoming impatient with what they perceive to be unproductive discussion.

Reflectors prefer to learn by observing individuals and groups, and thinking about their experiences. They need time to reflect and deliberate on what is presented to them and are good at producing in-depth analyses and reports if they are not given tight deadlines (although without a deadline they may never produce anything!). They tend to learn less well when they are required to act as the leader and dislike role-playing in front of others in a group. They need time to prepare and resist being rushed or hurried.

Most people display a mixture of all four styles although one or two tend to be dominant. Educators tend to replicate their learning style preferences in the teaching styles they adopt. Sometimes a trainer and trainee will happen to share the same learning preferences; this can result in a harmonious educational partnership, although it risks a degree of over-comfort and possible collusion, which can potentially inhibit the development of the less preferred learning styles in the trainee. More visible educational difficulties can arise when there is a large mismatch in preferences between learner and teacher – for example, a strongly reflective trainer and an activist trainee can have quite different opinions on the best ways to learn.

Using the curriculum to plan learning

Although specialty registrars, as adult learners, should ultimately take charge of their learning, there are times when every adult learner needs to be given guidance and direction. This is often the case for specialty registrars at the start of their attachment in general practice, when many report feeling overwhelmed by the initial volume of learning needs they perceive without having sufficiently developed the skills required to prioritise and address them.

Once a specialty registrar has defined some initial learning needs, the next step is for them to prioritise these needs, formulate the more complex needs into learning outcomes, and plan out appropriate educational activities. Chapter 3, 'Learning the curriculum', in this guide has more details on using the curriculum to assist in this process.

The topic statements and core competences described in the curriculum form a useful framework for mapping out activities to ensure all the domains of general practice are considered (see *Appendix 1* for a matrix suitable for planning out learning activities according to the curriculum domains).

Spiral learning and the curriculum

Spiral learning involves revisiting the same areas of the curriculum on several occasions over time. This may mean reviewing individual statements, competencies or even individual learning outcomes more than once, each time focusing in greater depth and complexity. This is similar to an aircraft descending in a spiral as it prepares to land – the concept will be familiar to anyone who has been in a plane descending over London. As the plane repeatedly circles round, lower and lower each time, the familiar landmarks and buildings can be seen in increasing detail.

Each time an area of the curriculum is revisited, learners:

- Review what was previously learned
- Reinforce the recognition of important patterns (e.g. patterns of health and disease)
- Gain a greater awareness of what determines their decisions
- Expand their range of management options
- Achieve a more complex understanding (e.g. enabling them to tailor their responses to the individual patient and to offer greater choice).

Developing teaching skills

GPs, as lifelong learners and educators, may become involved in leading a variety of educational activities throughout their career. These activities may include one-on-one tutorials, group teaching, seminars, workshops and presentations, all of which require different teaching styles and techniques. Developing a range of teaching styles can help educators engage more successfully with their learners and improve the effectiveness of the teaching. Successful educators develop the ability to choose from a wide range of teaching styles, according to the situation.

Table 4.4

Teaching methods and roles

Method	Process	Role of the teacher	Relevant authors
Didactic	Telling	Passing on knowledge	Many authors
Socratic	Questioning	Facilitating learning through awareness-raising questions	(Neighbour 1992)[10]
Heuristic	Encouraging	Promoting learner autonomy and self-directed learning	(Kolb 1984)[11] (Knowles 1990)[12] (Brookfield 1986)[13]
Counselling	Exploring	Encouraging self-awareness, self-discovery and reflective practice through exploring feelings and examining assumptions by using discussion and judicious challenge	(Schön 1987)[14] (Heron 1990)[15] (Bolton 2001)[16]

Source: RCGP curriculum statement 3.7: *Teaching, Mentoring and Clinical Supervision.*

GPs in training benefit hugely from opportunities to develop their own teaching and mentoring skills. This may include presenting to their colleagues, supervising medical students or teaching other health professionals. All GP educators (i.e. trainers, course organisers, programme directors, mentors, tutors or teachers) should be willing to receive feedback on their teaching skills; this will improve their performance and also encourages specialty registrars to adopt a similar critical approach to their own educational and professional skills.

Using the curriculum as a teaching resource

The curriculum statements themselves can be used as learning materials to resource a range of educational activities. In addition to the learning outcomes and knowledge base sections, the individual statements include a considerable amount of background info and point to some useful sources of further information. As such, curriculum statements form a useful basis for a comprehensive tutorial on a topic.

Table 4.5

Leading a teaching session based on a curriculum statement

A ten-point teaching plan:

1. Start the session and establish rapport with the learner(s)

2. Identify the learners' agenda and the teacher's agenda

3. Review the key messages, rationale and UK priorities described in the *acknowledgements* and *introduction* sections of the statement

4. Clarify the main issues and set them in the context of everyday practice

5. Explore the learners' suggestions, challenge preconceptions and give feedback

6. Clarify and record any learning needs that arise

7. Review the competencies and learning outcomes described for each of the curriculum domains in the *learning outcomes* section of the statement

8. Identify any unmet learning outcomes

9. Plan future learning activities

10. Summarise and conclude the session.

A list of common GP topics (for educational activities) and their corresponding curriculum statements is included in *Appendix 2* of this book.

Using the curriculum to address training difficulties

The curriculum is a competency-based document and has been designed to support the training needs of all GPs. It is a useful tool in addressing common problems that specialty registrars may run into. At one extreme, this might involve assisting a trainer in supporting a trainee who is generally underperforming and, at the other extreme, using the curriculum to stretch the abilities of a high achiever.

Table 4.6

Using the curriculum to address training issues

The training issue	How to use the curriculum
A specialty registrar who is generally underperforming	1. Evaluate the specialty registrar's performance against the six core competences described in statement 1: *Being a General Practitioner* 2. Give constructive feedback 3. Think holistically – is there an external explanation for why the trainee is not performing well? 4. Identify learning needs and priorities 5. Use a spiral learning approach – start by focusing on the basic knowledge needs, then on applying the knowledge in practice, then on practising the more complex skills and finally on developing expertise
A specialty registrar having difficulty with a specific competency or task	1. Identify the competency (or everyday task) where the specific difficulty arises 2. Define the learning outcomes that together are required to perform that specific competency 3. Identify if the problem is related to a lack of knowledge, skill, or an attitudinal issue 4. Plan targeted learning activities to address the specific outcome(s) identified
A specialty registrar who is performing well and needs to be challenged further	1. Review a topic-based curriculum statement in depth with the registrar 2. Observe how the specialty registrar adapts his or her generic skills to the specific context covered by the statement 3. Consider each of the core competences and essential application features in turn 4. Give constructive feedback 5. Identify further learning needs and priorities

The role of feedback and formative assessment in training

Formative assessment (an evaluation of learning in progress) and summative assessment (an evaluation of what has been learned) are well-established processes in GP education. Some of the Workplace-Based Assessment tools in the new MRCGP are intended to perform both of these functions simultaneously.

This allows the trainer to assess previous learning and forms a useful framework for providing feedback to trainees on how they may improve their performance. You can find more details on the Workplace-Based Assessment in Chapter 5, 'Succeeding at the new MRCGP'.

A range of educational activities can provide a platform for providing constructive feedback, including:

- Random and problem case analysis
- Case-based discussion tool (part of the Workplace-Based Assessment)
- Reviewing a learner's portfolio, logbooks or reflective diary
- Video consultations (or listening in on phone consultations)
- Joint or shared surgeries.

The Pendleton feedback rules[17] can be useful for formal feedback activities, such as those undertaken for Workplace-Based Assessment, and are particularly helpful for those who are uncomfortable with giving or receiving feedback. It offers a useful model for people who tend to be overly self-critical as it forces them to describe what is positive about their behaviour or performance:

1. The learner performs the activity

2. Questions are allowed on points of clarification of fact

3. The learner describes what they did well

4. The person giving feedback says what they thought was done well

5. The learner describes what was not done so well and what could be done better

6. The person giving feedback says what they thought was not done so well and in a supportive manner suggests ways for improvement.

Table 4.7

Principles of constructive feedback

Principle	Example
Describe the behaviour you have observed rather than your own interpretation	'You didn't maintain eye contact with the patient and spoke in rather a flat tone', rather than: 'You seemed bored and uninterested'
Describe specific examples	'You arrived late for your morning surgery on three occasions last week', rather than: 'You're always turning up late for everything'
Remain non-judgemental	'It has been noticed that sometimes you don't reply when the reception staff say good morning', rather than: 'The staff think you are rude and unfriendly'

References

1   Fraser A, Thomas H, Deighan M, Davison I, *et al.* Directions for change: a national survey of general practice training in the United Kingdom *Education for Primary Care* 2007; **18(1)**: 23–4.

2   Senge P M. *The Fifth Discipline: the art and practice of the learning organization* New York: Doubleday Currency, 1990.

3   Swanwick T and Chana N. Workplace assessment for licensing in general practice *British Journal of General Practice* 2005; **55**: 461–7.

4   Lave J and Wenger E. *Situated Learning: legitimate peripheral participation* Cambridge: Cambridge University Press, 1991.

5   Mohanna K, Wall D, Chambers R. *Teaching Made Easy* Oxford: Radcliffe Medical Press, 2003.

6   Middleton P and Field S J. *The GP Trainer's Handbook* Oxford: Radcliffe Medical Press, 2001.

7   *Rating Scales for Vocational Training in General Practice*. Occasional Paper 40. London: RCGP, 1989.

8   Eve R. Meeting educational needs in general practice – learning with PUNs and DENs *Education for General Practice* 2000; **11**: 73–9.

9   www.peterhoney.com [accessed June 2007].

10 Neighbour R. *The Inner Apprentice* Newbury: Petroc, 1992.

11 Kolb D. *Experiential Learning* New Jersey: Prentice Hall, 1984.

12 Knowles M. *The Adult Learner: a neglected species.* Fourth edn. Houston: Gulf Publishing, 1990.

13 Brookfield S D. *Understanding and Facilitating Adult Learning* San Francisco: Jossey-Bass, 1986.

14 Schön D. *Educating the Reflective Practitioner* San Francisco: Jossey-Bass, 1987.

15 Heron J. *Helping the Client: a creative practical guide* London: Sage Publications Ltd, 1990.

16 Bolton G. *Reflective Practice: writing and professional development* London: Paul Chapman Publishing, 2001.

17 Pendleton D, Schofield T, Tate P, Havelock P. *The Consultation: an approach to teaching and learning* Oxford: Oxford Medical Publications, 1984.

5 Succeeding at the new MRCGP

The new MRCGP assessments

Until 2007 there were two sets of assessments that GP trainees would take to become a qualified GP at the end of their training. One was to complete the summative assessment process, involving an MCQ exam, an audit, a video (or simulated surgery) and a structured trainer's report. The other was to pass the four components of the MRCGP exam. Since September 2007, these two routes have been replaced with a single compulsory 'new MRCGP' assessment.

The new MRCGP assessment has three components:

1. **Applied Knowledge Test**
   A multiple-choice question paper

2. **Clinical Skills Assessment**
   An OSCE-style assessment of GP skills

3. **Workplace-Based Assessment**
   A continuous assessment based on an enhanced trainer's report.

This chapter describes some of the historical background to the new MRCGP assessments (useful if you want to understand why you are doing the assessments!), what the three components involve and how to complete them successfully.

The MRCGP and summative assessment – a brief history

The *MRCGP examination* was born in 1965 and became compulsory for GPs seeking entry into membership of the College in 1968. Since then, the examination has continued to evolve to the present-day modular 'new MRCGP' of the Modernising Medical Careers era. It has developed just as the discipline of general practice has developed and as assessment methodologies have become more sophisticated. The changing examination has reflected advances in clinical practice, the growing expectations of patients, changing political demands and the constant change in the administrative framework of primary care.

Summative assessment was introduced for all GP registrars completing their training in September 1996. This was the first introduction of a national assessment package for general practice and one of the biggest changes in vocational training in the UK. Its most important function was to identify incompetent doctors and therefore to protect patients from harm.

It must be remembered that summative assessment was a test of minimal competency in the wide range of knowledge, skills and attitudes required of an independent GP – there was evidence that the system that preceded summative assessment did not effectively identify incompetent doctors,[1] and the public wanted reassurance that only doctors who had achieved an agreed minimum standard of competence should be able to enter the profession. The vast majority of GP registrars, therefore, had no difficulty in passing summative assessment and increasing numbers began to take the MRCGP examination to prove that they had reached an optimum rather than minimum standard.

Summative assessment had four key components: an audit project, an assessment of videotaped consultations, a test of factual knowledge (multiple-choice questions); and a Structured Trainer's Report.[2] The GP trainer completed the report over the course of the trainee's year in general practice, to document that the trainee had demonstrated the core skills required to be a competent GP. The old MRCGP had four components: a written paper; a multiple-choice paper; a consultation skills assessment (by video submission or simulated surgery); and an oral examination.

Over time, as more doctors opted to take the MRCGP exam, the two assessments grew closer together, resulting in the creation of a single route for the assessment of the videotaped consultations, slightly reducing the burden of the assessment for trainees and their trainers.

The development of the new MRCGP assessments

While the new curriculum for GP training was being developed, the RCGP also started to work on its cousin, the new MRCGP assessment. The new MRCGP was introduced in August 2007, following approval by the Postgraduate Medical Education and Training Board (PMETB).[3] Unlike the old MRCGP, the new assessments are delivered in partnership with local deaneries, the regional bodies responsible for organising GP training.

The new MRCGP involves a combination of a Workplace-Based Assessment (WPBA), which covers the whole three years of GP training, and two nationally delivered assessments – the Clinical Skills Assessment (CSA) and the Applied Knowledge Test (AKT). Together, these three new assessments have replaced the old summative assessment system and old MRCGP exams.

The new MRCGP competency areas

The new MRCGP assessments are designed to assess GPs in training against 12 new competency areas (see Table 5.1).

Table 5.1

The 12 new MRCGP competency areas

The MRCGP assessments have been designed around 12 competency areas, also referred to as assessment domains, which represent the important aspects of general practice that can be appropriately assessed:

1 Communication and consultation skills
This includes how a GP communicates with patients and uses recognised consultation models and communication techniques.

2 Practising holistically
This considers the ability of the doctor to operate in physical, psychological, socio-economic and cultural dimensions, taking into account feelings as well as thoughts.

3 Data gathering and interpretation
This involves gathering and using data for making clinical judgements, the choice of physical examinations and investigations, and how they are interpreted.

4 Making a diagnosis/making decisions
This examines how a GP adopts a structured, conscious approach to decision making.

5 Clinical management
This assesses how a doctor recognises and manages common medical conditions in primary care.

6 Managing medical complexity and promoting health
This looks at the aspects of care that go beyond managing straightforward problems, including the management of co-morbidity, uncertainty, risk and approaches to health rather than just illness.

7 Primary-care administration and IMT
This includes the appropriate use of primary-care administration systems, effective record keeping and information technology for the benefit of patient care.

8 Working with colleagues and in teams
GPs must be able to work effectively with other health professionals to ensure good patient care, including the sharing of information with colleagues.

9 Community orientation
This involves managing the health and social care of the practice population and local community.

Continued over

10 Maintaining performance, learning and teaching

This looks at how doctors maintain their performance and ensure effective continuing professional development of themselves and others.

11 Maintaining an ethical approach to practice

This examines how GPs ensure they practice ethically, with integrity and a respect for diversity.

12 Fitness to practise

The GP's awareness of when his or her own performance, conduct or health, or that of others, might put patients at risk and the actions taken to protect patients.

The WPBA includes assessment of the important psychomotor skills (the clinical and practical skills specific to general practice). The CSA may also test a sample of these skills in the clinical stations.

How the new MRCGP assessments relate to the curriculum

The curriculum describes the core knowledge, skills and attitudes required to be a competent GP. However, measuring all these qualities in a way that is accurate, reliable and valid is not a straightforward task. It is not easy, for example, to reliably measure a GP trainee's true attitudes towards a patient – to do so would require considerable mind-reading skill, which is an ability that few GP trainers possess.[i]

It is quite possible, on the other hand, to reliably assess a trainee's behaviour and evaluate how he or she performs as a working GP. For this reason, the 12 new MRCGP competency areas focus on the *behaviours* a GP is expected to perform in the workplace. These behaviours are based directly on the six domains of competence and the three essential application features described in the curriculum. The relationship between the curriculum and the new MRCGP competency areas is shown in Table 5.2.

The new MRCGP syllabus

A new MRCGP syllabus has also been created as an appendix to the curriculum. This provides a summary of the knowledge, skills, attitudes and other attributes that will be tested in the new MRCGP assessments. The new syllabus is available on the RCGP curriculum website: www.rcgp-curriculum.org.uk.

Much of the content of the new MRCGP syllabus is taken from the knowledge base contained within the curriculum, from which it has been derived. The syllabus also contains some additional clinical topics, however, which are not currently covered by an

---

i Although many of them can do a good job of convincing you otherwise.

Table 5.2

The curriculum and the new MRCGP assessments

The RCGP curriculum	The new MRCGP assessments
The curriculum represents the knowledge, skills, attitudes and expertise required to be a GP. There are *32 curriculum statements*: one core statement that describes the core competences and essential features, and 31 topic statements that cover specific areas of general practice and put the core competences into context	The assessments have been designed to represent the key aspects of general practice that can be *assessed* but are not designed to represent the entirety of general practice on their own *The three new MRCGP components*: 1. The Applied Knowledge Test 2. The Clinical Skills Assessment 3. The Workplace-Based Assessment

The curriculum	Related MRCGP competency areas
• Primary-care management	• Clinical management • Working with colleagues and in teams • Primary-care administration and IM&T
• Person-centred care	• Communication & consulting skills
• Specific problem-solving skills	• Data gathering and interpretation • Making a diagnosis/making decisions
• A comprehensive approach	• Managing medical complexity
• Community orientation	• Community orientation
• A holistic approach	• Practising holistically
• Contextual features	• Community orientation*
• Attitudinal features	• Maintaining an ethical approach to practice • Fitness to practise
• Scientific features	• Maintaining performance, learning and teaching
• Psychomotor skills	• Tested by the CSA and WPBA
• Knowledge base	• Tested by the AKT

* The community orientation competency relates to two curriculum domains.

existing curriculum statement – examples include renal medicine and haematology. We have listed these 'missing' topics in condensed statement 15.X: *The rest of general practice* in Chapter 7, 'The essential knowledge'.

Chapter 7 also includes all the condensed statements, which contain the key items of knowledge and the practical skills included in the curriculum's knowledge base and makes a useful revision guide when preparing for the new MRCGP assessments.

Getting to grips with the new MRCGP

The new MRCGP has three components:

1. **Applied Knowledge Test**
   A multiple-choice question paper

2. **Clinical Skills Assessment**
   An OSCE-style assessment of GP skills

3. **Workplace-Based Assessment**
   A continuous assessment based on an enhanced trainer's report.

The new *MRCGP* assessments are considerably more sophisticated than their predecessors and a considerable amount of information is available to explain the three assessments in detail from the RCGP. Much of this information is fairly technical and many trainees and educators may not be familiar with some of the new terminology that has been adopted. In particular, a large number of tools and assessments now exist, many of which are referred to by an acronym. To help you get to grips with these, you may find it useful to refer to our *new MRCGP acronym-buster* in Table 5.3.

The Applied Knowledge Test

The Applied Knowledge Test or AKT is a multiple-choice question paper, which will be marked by computer. There are around 200 items in the test, which must be completed in three hours. There will be three types of questions:

1. Extended matching questions

Each question consists of a scenario that has to be matched to an answer from a list of possible options. There may be several possible answers but you must choose only the most likely answer from the list of options. This may represent the single most likely diagnosis or the *single most appropriate statement* that matches the scenario.

Table 5.3

The new MRCGP acronym-buster!

The new MRCGP suffers from an epidemic of TFLAs – three- and four-letter acronyms. Here are what some of the commonly used acronyms stand for:

AKT	Applied Knowledge Test
CBD	Case-based discussion
CEX	Clinical evaluation exercise
COT	Consultation observation tool
CSA	Clinical Skills Assessment
CSR	Clinical Supervisor's Report
DOPS	Direct observation of procedural skills
EMQ	Extended matching question
MCQ	Multiple-choice question
MMC	Modernising Medical Careers
MSF	Multi-source feedback
MTAS	Medical Training Application Service
OSCE	Objective structured clinical examination
PSQ	Patient satisfaction questionnaire
RITA	Record of in-training assessment
SBA	Single best answer questions
WPBA	Workplace-Based Assessment

Table 5.4

An example of the extended matching question style[ii]

Option list:

A Eczema

B Psoriasis

C Herpes simplex

D Scabies

E *Molluscum contagiosum*

F Cutaneous larva migrans

Instruction:

For each patient described below, select the *single most likely* diagnosis. Each option may be used once, more than once, or not at all.

Items:

1 A 45-year-old man presents with thickened red plaques with a silvery scale on the extensor surfaces of his knees and elbows

2 A 5-year-old girl has developed a small cluster of umbilicated pearly papules on her chest, but is otherwise well

3 A 19-year-old student attends with a widespread, excoriated rash on his arms, trunk and groin, which is intensely itchy, especially at night. Examination of his wrist reveals several small, irregular track-like marks

2. Single best answer questions

This is a common multiple-choice question format. Each question consists of a statement or stem followed by a number of options, only one of which is correct.

---

ii The MCQ examples included here are intended to demonstrate the style of question and are not official new MRCGP exam questions.

Table 5.5

An example of a single best answer question style

*Which **ONE** of the following is a recommended first-line treatment for menorrhagia?*
Select one option only.

A	Mefenamic acid
B	The combined oral contraceptive pill
C	Endometrial ablation
D	Levonorgestrel-releasing intrauterine system
E	Hysterectomy

3. Table/algorithm completion

These questions are similar to the algorithm layout often found in guidelines that provide advice on management decisions. The candidate must select the answer that correctly completes the table, flowchart or algorithm.

Preparing for the Applied Knowledge Test

The AKT tests both clinical and non-clinical aspects of general practice knowledge and assesses the application of knowledge, including decision making, evaluation of evidence and undifferentiated problems, and decisions regarding patient safety. The questions are based on the knowledge contained within the RCGP curriculum and new MRCGP syllabus, distributed as follows:

- Clinical medicine (80%)
- Administration and health informatics (10%)
- Research, critical appraisal, evidence-based medicine and statistics (10%).

The questions in the AKT relate to current best practice rather than local arrangements and so answers should be based on published evidence. Because some experience of real-life general practice is required, it is advised that trainees do not attempt the AKT until they have worked in general practice for at least two to three months. The AKT is offered three times a year at centres across the UK so trainees are able to attempt it up to three times in a 12-month training period.

Questions are derived from accredited and referenced sources. These include review articles and original papers from well-known journals and resources, including: *Clinical Evidence, British Medical Journal*, NICE guidelines, *British Journal of General Practice, Drugs and Therapeutics Bulletin* and *Cochrane Review*. Questions on therapeutics and prescribing will be based on information from the *British National Formulary*. Many of these journals and publications are available free of charge to RCGP members and associates in training (specialty registrars) via the RCGP website: www.rcgp.org.uk.

One of the best ways of preparing for the AKT is by ensuring you have a broad working knowledge of general practice, as described in the curriculum. We have extracted the core knowledge and skills from each of the curriculum statements in Chapter 7, 'The essential knowledge'. Doing lots of practice MCQs can also be a highly effective way to prepare for the exam, although it is not the most inspiring way to learn general practice.

Table 5.6

Tips for preparing for the Applied Knowledge Test	
Practice MCQs	The AKT is new but there are lots of MCQ books available that cover the old MRCGP MCQ paper. A number of new books have also been published recently to support preparation for the AKT. PLAB books often include extended matching questions
Learning modules	Doctors.net (www.doctors.net.uk) and BMJ Learning (www.bmjlearning.com) offer learning modules that contain MCQs and extended matching questions. GPNotebook (www.gpnotebook.co.uk) offers educational modules ('GEMS') on the key clinical topics that are useful for revision
PEP eKit	RCGP Scotland has produced an interactive e-learning resource including MCQs on a range of clinical topics[iii]
Critical appraisal workbooks	Several books are available that offer data interpretation questions (e.g. interpreting ECGs, spirometry, audiometry)

The Clinical Skills Assessment

The Clinical Skills Assessment or CSA takes the form of an OSCE-style examination with 13 stations, each lasting 10 minutes, and tests clinical, communication and practical skills. It is based on simulated consultations with specially trained actors playing the role of patients. Candidates undertake a mock 'surgery' and

iii Available at: www.pep-ekit.org.uk.

will remain at their station throughout the assessment while the simulated patients and examiners rotate around them.

Each candidate's performance is graded as clear pass, marginal pass, marginal fail or clear fail. The examiners are fully trained and experienced MRCGP assessors, and all candidates receive feedback on their performance. The CSA is currently only available at one centre and takes place three times a year, during a three- or four-week period in February, May and October.

Preparing for the Clinical Skills Assessment

The purpose of the CSA is to assess doctors' ability to bring together and apply their clinical, professional, communication and practical skills to a standard appropriate for general practice. It has been designed to focus on core GP skills that can be assessed outside the practice to an agreed national standard (to reduce any distortion that might be introduced by individual trainer and local deanery variation).

Table 5.7

Aspects of general practice covered by the Clinical Skills Assessment	
Primary care management	Recognising and managing common medical conditions in primary care
Problem-solving skills	Gathering and using data for clinical judgement, choice of examination, investigations and their interpretation. Demonstration of a structured and flexible approach to decision making
Comprehensive approach	Demonstrating proficiency in the management of co-morbidity and risk
Person-centred approach	Communicating with patient and using recognised consultation techniques to promote a shared approach to managing problems
Attitudinal aspects	Practising ethically with respect for equality and diversity, with accepted professional codes of conduct
Psychomotor skills (clinical and practical skills)	Demonstrating proficiency in performing physical examinations and using diagnostic and therapeutic instruments

Patient safety is also an important aspect of the Clinical Skills Assessment – one of the key functions of the CSA is to identify GPs who put patients at risk.

It is recommended that trainees gain at least six months of general practice experience before attempting the CSA. It is estimated that around 20 per cent of GP trainees may have to take the CSA twice in order to pass, and 10 per cent three times. Trainees who fail the CSA three times will be offered extra support to look further into why this has occurred; it may be that certain factors in the trainee's learning environment need to be addressed.

Stations that might come up in the CSA include:

- Communicating sensitively with a depressed patient (played by an actor) and assessing his or her suicide risk

- Checking and demonstrating the inhaler technique of a patient with asthma

- Demonstrating how to perform a vaginal examination on a manikin.

Table 5.8

Tips for preparing for the Clinical Skills Assessment	
Learning groups	Learning groups are particularly suitable for preparing for the 'softer' topics, including ethical and professional dilemmas
Mock CSA OSCEs and revision courses	Some local training programmes may offer practice OSCE stations and consultation scenarios. The high-quality preparation courses for the new MRCGP will include CSA practice stations
Skills simulator laboratories	'Skills simulator labs' are useful for learning new psychomotor skills and those not performed often in daily practice where gaining sufficient experience is otherwise difficult (e.g. minor surgical techniques, inserting catheters, Basic Life Support skills)
Log of procedures	Keep a log of the procedures you undertake – this should form part of the Workplace-Based Assessment. Make sure you are competent in all the psychomotor skills described in the essential knowledge (e.g. arrange to spend time with a practice nurse or HCA doing ECGs or spirometry then tick off in the book when you are confident)
Consultation analysis	Video lots of consultations and review them – use a variety of methods to analyse them (see the essential knowledge – statement 2: *The General Practice Consultation*). Watch videos with different GPs, your trainer or mentor, other GPs in the practice, your course organisers and your learning group (bearing in mind patient confidentiality and that you must obtain informed consent). Don't worry if you cringe at first when watching yourself consulting – this is entirely normal!

Joint surgeries	Analyse a range of healthcare professionals' consulting styles (e.g. sit in, or watch a video they have made). What do they do well? What could they do better? You can learn lots from observing the tricks and techniques used successfully by other people
Role-play	Like sprouts at Christmas, role-play is one of those things you just have to do. It can be done with your peers, your trainer, and other members of staff or even professional actors. Always bear in mind the rules of giving effective feedback and be sensitive until you are certain that everyone present is comfortable with giving and receiving feedback
360° feedback	Encourage colleagues to give feedback on your management of patients – this can be useful when they subsequently see a patient you found challenging. What approach did they find successful?

The Workplace-Based Assessment

The RCGP curriculum emphasises the importance of learning in the workplace and this is reflected in the Workplace-Based Assessment (WPBA) component of the new MRCGP.[4] This assessment is designed to bring teaching, learning and assessment together into one continuing process; trainees gather evidence of their actual performance in the workplace, which enables those aspects of professional behaviour that cannot be tested reliably outside the practice to be assessed, such as time management and team-working.

The WPBA is designed around an enhanced trainer's report. This requires the trainee to maintain a Training Record (TR) to house a portfolio of evidence that enables the trainer to judge the trainee's progress and give feedback in each of the 12 MRCGP competency areas.

The e-portfolio

An electronic portfolio has been specially developed to enable every specialty registrar and trainer to collect all the evidence they need to complete the Workplace-Based Assessment. The e-portfolio stores the trainee's *Training Record*, which contains:

- **The evidence of competency**
  The trainee's progress in the 12 MRCGP competency areas is recorded at regular intervals when the evidence of performance is regularly reviewed (see below)

- **A record of learning**
  Learning activities can be recorded (e.g. tutorials, group learning, seminars) and stored under the relevant curriculum statement heading

- **A technical skills log**
  Examination skills and procedures undertaken (e.g. joint injections, minor ops) can be recorded along with the direct observation of procedural skills assessment (DOPS).
       An e-portfolio is made available to every trainee when they begin their three-year training programme.

Collecting the evidence and using the WPBA tools

Much of the evidence for the Workplace-Based Assessment is intended to be 'naturally occurring' and can be collected informally. Assessment tools have been specially developed for gathering evidence both within the practice and externally. Some of these tools are mandatory (i.e. every trainee must complete them) whereas others are optional.

The following two assessment tools are *mandatory* and are *externally moderated*:

- **Multi-source feedback (MSF)**
  This is a web-based tool designed to collect and evaluate feedback from peers and colleagues

- **Patient satisfaction questionnaire (PSQ)**
  This is designed to collect and evaluate feedback from patients.

The following two assessment tools are also *mandatory* and are designed for use *within the practice*:

- **Case-based discussion (CBD)**
  This is a structured interview designed to assess the GP trainee's clinical and professional judgement in cases selected for discussion by the trainer or trainee

- **Consultation observation tool (COT)**
  This is a tool designed to help trainers assess videoed consultations, and is based on the previous summative assessment and old MRCGP video criteria.

The Workplace-Based Assessment continues throughout the entire three-year GP training period. To review their progress during their hospital posts, trainees undergo six-monthly reviews with their secondary-care clinical supervisor (e.g. a consultant) and a trainer. During this process, the trainee's clinical supervisor completes a Clinical Supervisor's Report (CSR). Reviews carried out in secondary care make use of the following validated tools:[iv]

- **Mini-clinical evaluation exercise (mini-CEX)**
  This is a validated case-based discussion tool and is used in place of the consultation observation tool (COT) while the GP trainee is working in secondary care

- **Direct observation of procedural skills (DOPS)**
  This is a tool for assessing the GP trainee's clinical skills.

Table 5.9

Tools for collecting evidence for the Workplace-Based Assessment

MRCGP competency area	MSF	PSQ	COT	CBD	CEX	CSR
Communication and consultation skills	☑	☑	☑		☑	☑
Practising holistically		☑	☑	☑		☑
Data gathering and interpretation	☑		☑	☑	☑	☑
Making a diagnosis/making decisions	☑		☑	☑	☑	☑
Clinical management	☑		☑	☑	☑	☑
Managing medical complexity				☑	☑	☑
Primary-care administration and IMT				☑		
Working with colleagues and in teams	☑			☑		☑
Community orientation				☑		☑
Maintaining performance, learning and teaching	☑				☑	☑
Maintaining an ethical approach	☑			☑		☑
Fitness to practise	☑			☑		☑

A number of additional optional assessment tools are available for the trainer and trainee to use to gather evidence of performance. It is not compulsory to use all the tools available but trainees will need to make sufficient use of them to enable the collection of enough evidence to complete the various parts of the WPBA:

- Videos of consultations

- Practice audit

- Significant event analysis

iv Further details of these tools can be found on the RCGP website (www.rcgp.org.uk) and the assessment section of the NHS Modernising Medical Careers website (www.mmc.nhs.uk).

- Referrals and prescribing analysis.

The six-monthly interim review

At six-month intervals, every specialty registrar meets with his or her trainer (and his or her educational supervisor/consultant while in secondary care) to undertake an interim review of his or her progress and current performance. The evidence the trainee has collected to date is reviewed, a self-assessment completed and the trainee's progress evaluated by the trainer in each of the 12 assessment domains.

This review process involves:

- Reviewing the evidence of achievement
- Making a judgement of performance[v]
- Giving feedback
- Setting educational goals and objectives
- Planning the next phase of training.

Table 5.10

Timetable for collecting the required evidence for the WPBA[5]

Specialty Training Year 1	Specialty Training Year 2	Specialty Training Year 3
For the six-month review:	**For the 18-month review:**	**For the 30-month review (in primary care):**
• 3 × COT or mini-CEX • 3 × CBD • 1 × MSF (five clinicians only) • DOPS* • Clinical supervisor's report*	• 3 × COT or mini-CEX • 3 × CBD • PSQ,+ if not completed in ST1 • DOPS* • Clinical supervisor's report* +only if in primary care	• 6 × CBD • 6 × COT • 1 × MSF
*only if in secondary care	*only if in secondary care	
For the 12-month review:	**For the 24-month review:**	**For the 34-month review:**
• 3 × COT or mini-CEX • 3 × CBD • 1 × MSF (five clinicians only) • 1 × PSQ+ • DOPS* • Clinical supervisor's report*	• 3 × COT or mini-CEX • 3 × CBD • PSQ,+ if not completed in ST1 • DOPS* • Clinical supervisor's report*	• 6 × CBD • 6 × COT • 1 × MSF • 1 × PSQ
+only if in primary care *only if in secondary care	+only if in primary care *only if in secondary care	

Notes

1. COT is used in primary care and mini-CEX in secondary care

2. DOPS is not repeated once the mandatory practical skills have been assessed as satisfactory

3. Patient satisfaction is assessed only in primary care

4. Multi-source feedback involves clinicians only when in secondary care and both clinicians and non-clinicians in primary care.

The final review

Shortly before the end of the three-year training period, a final summative review is carried out. At this point, trainers make a recommendation to their local deanery regarding the compe-tency of their specialty registrars. To complete training success-fully, the specialty registrar must have demonstrated aptitude in all 12 of the new MRCGP competency areas. Failure to reach the required standard triggers a review by a panel of experts in the local deanery, which then judges whether the WPBA has been completed satisfactorily.

v Similar to a RITA (record of in-training assessment).

As the WPBA involves the evaluation of a trainee's progress over three years of training, it cannot be completed early and will only be signed off in the final period of the third year. The judgements made by the trainers on the standard of the trainees will be externally moderated by their local deanery, which will review all the evidence that has been collected, including the evidence gathered from the externally moderated assessments.

Once the WPBA and the other assessments have been completed, successful specialty registrars can apply for their Certificate of Completion of Training and have their name added to the GP register – then the really hard work begins!

References

1 Campbell L M and Murray T S. Summative assessment of vocational trainees: results of a 3-year study *British Journal of General Practice* 1996; **46**: 441–4.

2 www.nosa.org.uk [accessed June 2007].

3 www.pmetb.org.uk [accessed June 2007].

4 Swanwick T, Williams N, Evans A. Workplace assessment for the licensing of general practitioners: a qualitative pilot study of a competency-based trainer's report *Education for Primary Care* 2006; **17**: 5.

5 www.rcgp.org.uk [accessed June 2007].

Part II

The condensed curriculum

In the following sections of the book, we have condensed the curriculum down to a fraction of its original size. We have done this by separating the key educational content into its two main ingredients – *the core competences* and *the essential knowledge*.

How we condensed the curriculum

The curriculum is a large and wide-ranging document. In all, it contains 32 separate statements, about 500 pages of text and over 1350 learning outcomes. Each of the 32 statements spells out how the core GP competences, as described in statement 1: *Being a General Practitioner*, are applied to each topic or patient group. This makes the statements very comprehensive and holistic educational tools – a statement is a great resource for learning or teaching about a particular area of general practice – but means that altogether the statements contain a considerable amount of repetition.

The condensed curriculum is not meant to replace the full RCGP curriculum, but to represent its key messages and important educational content. This is intended to make the curriculum content easily accessible to GP learners and teachers, and enables readers to gain an overall understanding of how to learn and teach the core knowledge and skills central to general practice.

6 The core competences

The core competences of general practice

The first statement of the curriculum, *Being a General Practitioner*, describes the core knowledge, skills, attitudes and expertise a doctor needs to acquire to become a competent GP. For this reason it is known as the core statement. 'Core' means that it is essential to general practice, irrespective of the healthcare system in which it takes place.

The six core competences and the three essential application features of the curriculum put the core of general practice into a framework that allows it to be learned. This chapter explains exactly what these core competences and essential features mean, and gives some suggestions on how to learn them.

How the core competences were identified

Before the curriculum was created, several documents had been written that defined the *generic* competencies of a doctor. These generic competencies are the professional abilities and attributes that are expected of every doctor, regardless of his or her specialty.

The publication *Good Medical Practice*,[1] produced by the General Medical Council (GMC), provides a framework for judging the performance of all doctors. After an edition of this document was published in 2001, the RCGP and the General Practitioners Committee of the British Medical Association tweaked it to make it more specific to general practice, leading to the publication of *Good Medical Practice for General Practitioners*.[2] Each of the statements in the curriculum has been mapped to this document to make sure all of the generic professional competencies have been covered.

As well as covering the generic competencies expected of every doctor, the curriculum covers the core competences that are specific to performing as a GP. The core curriculum statement, *Being a General Practitioner*, is based on the framework for general practice produced by WONCA Europe.[3] This was endorsed by the RCGP and the Joint Committee on Postgraduate Training for General Practice (JCPTGP)[i] and it subsequently became the framework for the entire RCGP curriculum.

---

i The JCPTGP ceased to exist in 2005 when its responsibilities for regulating GP training were taken over by the Postgraduate Medical Education and Training Board (PMETB).

A quick overview of the core competences

The first three core competences focus mainly on the GP consultation:

1. Primary care management
This is managing the first contact with patients in primary care. It includes addressing people's unselected problems, coordinating care with other primary-care professionals and with specialists, providing appropriate care to patients in the practice and making effective use of the health service.

2. Person-centred care
This involves being able to establish an effective doctor–patient relationship that demonstrates respect for the patient's autonomy, an ability to set priorities and act in partnership with patients, providing continuity of care and coordinating care.

3. Specific problem-solving skills
This includes selective history taking, physical examinations and investigations, formulating an appropriate and effective management plan, dealing with conditions that present early on in the course of an illness and in an undifferentiated way, making diagnoses related to the incidence and prevalence of conditions in the community, using appropriate GP techniques such as 'time as a diagnostic tool' and 'tolerating uncertainty', spotting conditions or symptoms that may be serious and intervening urgently when required.

The remaining three core competences are more subtle and complex. Some may consider them to represent the 'woolly' aspects of general practice. They involve taking a wider perspective than just the immediate issues arising in the consultation:

4. A comprehensive approach
This involves mastering the skills to simultaneously manage multiple complaints and pathologies in one individual, managing both acute and chronic health problems that may coexist, successfully promoting health and implementing disease prevention strategies.

5. Community orientation
This requires the ability to reconcile the health needs of individual patients and the health needs of the community in which they live, taking account of the resources that are available.

6. A holistic approach

This involves caring for the whole person in the context of the person's values, their family beliefs, their family system, and their culture in the larger community, and considering a range of therapies based on the evidence of their benefits and cost. An understanding of our own limitations as GPs is essential because of the emphasis on the therapeutic partnership between GP and patient.

Our tips for learning and teaching the core competences

The following pages describe the core competences of general practice in detail. Each competence is divided into a number of professional tasks known as competencies,[ii] and each of these competencies is broken down further into individual learning outcomes.

With each learning outcome we have included relevant tips and suggestions for interpreting, learning or teaching that particular outcome. These tips are drawn from a variety of sources including the published literature, educational workshops, the advice of established trainers, course organisers, programme directors and other GP educationalists. The authors are all working GPs involved in education and have borrowed heavily from their own practical experience of learning, teaching, training and caring for patients in everyday general practice.

Is it knowledge, skill or attitude?

The learning outcomes that make up each competency can be categorised as an item of knowledge, skill or attitude. This is indicated by use of the letters *K*, *S* or *A* as appropriate.

---

ii Note the minor difference in spelling between competences and competencies, which can be a source of considerable confusion!

The six core competences

Competence 1 – primary care management

GPs work in the community, where the population has a lower prevalence of serious disease, so it is crucial that a GP understands concepts of health, function and quality of life, as well as disease. GPs play an important role in disease prevention and health promotion, risk management, and in palliative and terminal care. GPs also need to be conscious of healthcare costs and understand the concept of cost-efficiency.

Primary care involves working with a team of health professionals, both within the practice and in the local community, and also working with specialists in secondary care, so every GP must learn to integrate different disciplines within the complex team of the NHS. GPs must also learn the importance of supporting patients' decisions about the management of their health problems and communicating how their care will be delivered.

1.1 Managing primary contact with patients and dealing with unselected problems

What this involves

1.1a	**K** Knowledge of the epidemiology of problems presenting in primary care
Our tips	A GP should be familiar with how patients present in the early stages of illness and develop a good sense of which conditions are common and which conditions are rare. Similarly, a GP needs to be aware of which red-flag symptoms and signs may indicate a potentially serious condition and understand important risk factors and how these influence decisions on investigation and management.
	Here are some ways to learn about epidemiology in primary care:
	• Go through Chapter 7, 'The essential knowledge', which contains the common clinical conditions
	• Do computer searches of chronic disease in your practice population
	• Keep a log of patients you see to identify what problems tend to come up and how they first present
	• Review information published by reputable bodies (e.g. Cancer Research UK publishes cancer statistics: www.cancerresearchuk.org).

1.1b	**S Mastering an approach that allows easy access for patients with unselected problems**

Our tips	Patients rarely walk in saying, 'Doctor, I have a pulmonary embolism, what would you like to do about it?' Rather, they present with a collection of symptoms or concerns that may or may not fit familiar patterns. GPs must therefore develop a consulting style that enables them to rationalise unselected complaints and formulate an understanding of the key issues. To do this, GPs need to master eliciting and active listening skills, in order to obtain the relevant information they need, and summarising skills to check their understanding of the patient's ideas, concerns and expectations. GPs also need the ability to apply their medical knowledge appropriately to make sense of the patient's narrative, to decide whether to include or exclude the most important diagnoses and to formulate an appropriate management plan.
	The development of an effective consultation style takes time, experience and lots of practice. GPs who are particularly good at consulting tend to develop a flexible consulting style, adopting a range of approaches and techniques that can be put to use when needed, depending on the context of the consultation and the preferences of the individual patient.
	See 'The essential knowledge – statement 2: *The General Practice Consultation* for more advice and techniques on how to develop consultation skills.

1.1c	**S An organisational approach to the management of chronic conditions**

Our tips	Practices adopt different strategies for organising the management of patients with certain chronic conditions. In some practices, for example, chronic disease management of diabetes is carried out almost exclusively in nurse-led clinics, whereas in other practices patients with diabetes are managed in routine GP surgeries. GPs need to develop the appropriate skills to organise chronic disease management in their practice and work effectively with other primary-care team members.
	Ways to learn about the organisation of chronic disease management include:

- Finding out how chronic disease management is organised in your practice and in the practices of your colleagues – there is a surprising amount of variation between practices
- Attending or running a chronic disease management (CDM) clinic

- Reviewing your practice's protocols and computer templates (what does an annual diabetes or asthma check actually involve?)
- Auditing practice patient outcomes against recognised standards
- Reviewing the practice QoF data
- Discussion with the practice manager or nursing team leader about how a particular CDM clinic was set up and the issues encountered
- Reviewing your practice's chronic disease registers and identifying individual cases where you could become involved
- Obtaining feedback from patients attending the clinics.

1.1d	**K Knowledge of the conditions encountered in primary care and their treatment**
Our tips	There is a massive amount of potential knowledge for a GP to assimilate, as general practice is the broadest field of medicine. An essential skill for all GPs, therefore, is to learn how to identify individually what knowledge they do or do not need to learn in order to perform competently.
	The knowledge base contained within the curriculum statements describes a core syllabus of knowledge every GP should be familiar with (see Chapter 7, 'The essential knowledge'). This is a good basis for general practice although it is not all encompassing and the knowledge required of a working GP continually evolves over time and depends on individual circumstances.
	Here are some popular methods of identifying knowledge-based learning needs in general practice:

- Keep a log of learning needs arising from patients you see – a log is especially useful at the start of GP training when you want to remember to look up lots of straightforward pieces of information
- PUNS and DENS[4]
- The Johari window[5]
- Random and selected case analysis
- Confidence and competence rating scales
- Formative assessments
- Clinical questions logbook
- Practice exam questions and MCQs.

A range of educational tools to help identify learning needs are available on the RCGP curriculum website: www.rcgp-curriculum.org.uk.

Once you have identified your learning needs you need to formulate a system for recording them and your action plans – this can form the basis of your personal development plan. Resources that support learning and provide information are described in Chapter 7, 'The essential knowledge'.

1.2 Covering the full range of health conditions

What this involves

1.2a	**K Knowledge of preventive activities required in the practise of primary care**
Our tips	'Prevention is better than cure' – or at least it saves some of the work. Find out what preventive activities the practice participates in already (e.g. smoking cessation, men's/women's/teenage health clinics, sexual health screening). Is there any preventive activity important to the local population that the practice should be participating in but currently isn't? See below for how you can find this out.

1.2b	**S Skills in acute, chronic, preventive, palliative and emergency care**
Our tips	As you probably realise, the G in GP stands for general! A generalist must develop the skills required to deal with every problem that comes through the door – patients might arrive as 'worried well', 'ill but not too sick', 'very sick' or even 'about to drop dead' – and a competent GP must be able to react appropriately and implement appropriate initial management.
	GPs in training may find that it is hard for them to gain enough experience to feel comfortable about managing certain groups of patients by the time they start work in primary care. Some hospital jobs (e.g. acute medicine, A&E) can provide good emergency and acute illness experience, while others may provide a range of chronic disease experience (e.g. old-age medicine, community hospital jobs). If you are based in hospital, consider what opportunities exist in your current post for you to gain experience and which 'gaps' in experience you may wish to focus on in primary care.
	During the short time available for GP training in primary care, trainees may find their experience of caring for the terminally ill and dying is quite limited (which in some respects is a good thing). This important aspect of general practice can be addressed if properly planned from the start. Talk to your trainer about sharing the palliative care of a patient with his or her regular doctor, or arrange to spend some time with the Macmillan nurses. Some training schemes offer hospital jobs in palliative care departments and these may offer contacts who can provide useful advice.

1.2c	**S Clinical skills in history taking, physical examination and use of ancillary tests to diagnose conditions presented in primary care**
Our tips	Focused history and examination skills are key to being a GP – especially in the primary-care context where time is short and access to diagnostic tests is often limited. A GP needs to be able to elicit sufficient useful information to rapidly and accurately diagnose conditions, assess their severity and decide whether further investigations are indicated. The Clinical Skills Assessment (CSA) of the new MRCGP tests this important competency.
	Shared surgeries (preferably with a variety of experienced GPs) are very good for picking up useful consulting tips, gaining feedback on current performance and for bringing back complex patients for a more experienced opinion.

1.2d	**S Skills in therapeutics, including drug and non-drug approaches to treatment of conditions (in primary care)**
Our tips	A GP needs to become familiar with a repertoire of frequently used treatments (both drug and non-drug) and their indications, contraindications, and common or potentially serious side effects.
	There is an important element of being evidence-based in this learning outcome and monitoring the therapeutic interventions you initiate on an ongoing basis. As a working GP, you may quickly become comfortable with a select group of 'favourite' treatments – this should mean you are familiar with the risks and benefits but also risks making you inappropriately reluctant to use unfamiliar treatments that may have been shown to be more effective, or alternatively may make you reluctant to stop using treatments that are no longer recommended.
	A number of publications and information sources are available to aid treatment decisions. The *British National Formulary* (BNF) is obviously a key resource for medications and also includes information on some dressings and appliances. The *Drugs and Therapeutics Bulletin*, the BMJ's *Clinical Evidence* and websites such as NHS Clinical Knowledge Summaries (http://cks.library.nhs.uk) can also help guide treatment decisions. Your Primary Care Trust (PCT) will also issue local prescribing guidelines and your practice may have its own protocols and formulary.

1.2e	**S The ability to prioritise problems**
Our tips	There is a limit to how many things anyone can manage at one time – this applies both to the multiple problems of an individual patient and to the individual problems of multiple patients! Not forgetting your own non-clinical problems too!
	Some GPs attempt to impose a strict limit on the number of problems a patient is allowed to raise in a single consultation. This may be an attempt on the GP's part to compensate for deficiencies in his or her own ability to deal with multiple problems. As many patients may 'test out' their GP with a minor issue first before raising a greater concern, an inflexible approach risks spending the entire consultation on a trivial problem at the expense of a serious one.
	Other GPs take the approach that it is better to allow patients to list all their problems in detail and then deal with them all one-by-one in a single sitting. Long consultations produce higher patient satisfaction[6] but this unstructured approach may result in exhausting consultations and poor time-keeping.
	A third approach is to encourage the patient to briefly 'unpack' all his or her problems at the start of the consultation (when it will often become apparent that they are all linked to one underlying issue), and then discuss with the patient which problems it would be best to concentrate on, given the time available, and which it may be more appropriate to discuss at another time. In our own experience, this approach is usually the most successful, but it does require the GP to develop the ability to prioritise problems.
	One useful technique for prioritising multiple problems is to categorise them into *urgent* or *non-urgent* and then into *serious* or *less serious*. The urgent and serious problems should be addressed first, the urgent but less serious problems may be dealt with if time allows, the non-urgent but serious problems should be addressed properly at the appropriate time, and the non-urgent, less serious problems can be deferred (with appropriate safety-netting – as per Neighbour's five-checkpoint consultation model[7]). Obviously, the GP's and patient's view of what is urgent and what is serious may differ, and this is where good negotiation skills are required!

1.3 Coordinating care with other professionals in primary care, and with other specialties

What this involves

1.3a	**K** Knowing how NHS primary care is organised
Our tips	Firstly, find out who works in your practice and what their roles are, as a partner, a clinician or a member of staff. Ideally, this should be covered during an induction programme. Then, find out who is involved in the wider primary-care team that has direct contact with the practice (e.g. district nurses, health visitors, midwives, counsellors, physiotherapists).
	There is a whole range of wider health professionals who work in primary care (e.g. podiatrists, opticians, community pharmacists, specialist nurses, visiting consultants) and their roles vary from locality to locality. The local PCT and practice-based commissioning organisation will be able to provide you with up-to-date information on the primary-care services in your area.

1.3b	**K** Understanding the importance of excellent communication with patients and staff, and **S** skills in effective teamwork
Our tips	Being a GP increasingly requires the ability to be an effective team player and, when required, a team leader. We all know from experience that we find it easier to work with some people than with others. When asked, however, few people freely admit that they consider themselves a poor team player. The number of solo GPs is dwindling, and even they must work effectively on a daily basis with other health professionals.
	Formative team feedback (e.g. from a 360° appraisal) can be an extremely useful process for developing your teamwork skills. However, it is very important to make sure that this process is carried out sensitively, and until the individual concerned is familiar and secure with feedback (and aware of how team members may respond), it may be best for feedback to be collated by a mentor (e.g. a trainer, practice manager or appraiser) and discussed in a supportive environment. Team members giving feedback should be reminded to comment constructively on an individual's behaviour and not their personality.[8]

1.4 Mastering effective and appropriate care provision and health service utilisation

What this involves

1.4a	**K Knowledge of the structure of the healthcare system and the function of primary care within the wider NHS**

Our tips	The NHS is an ever-changing and increasingly complex organisation! Find out who is the most politically astute GP in the practice as they may be best placed to tell you all about the latest NHS reforms, future threats and opportunities, and the impact of political developments on your practice.
	Practice managers have considerable contact with other local NHS bodies and it may be worth arranging a tutorial with them to discuss these and other organisational developments, such as practice-based commissioning.[9] Other useful contacts include your local medical committee and PCT representatives. Your course organiser may be able to arrange one of these to resource a learning seminar on NHS organisation. The weekly GP newspapers and BMA website (www.bma.org.uk) contain lots of information on NHS changes affecting primary care.

1.4b	**K Understanding the processes of referral into secondary care and other care pathways**

Our tips	It is essential for GPs to be able to access appropriate care for their patients. There is currently a shift towards the provision of more care in the primary-care setting, and over the past decade the concept of patient care pathways has influenced how services are designed.[10]
	Some practices will keep a folder or maintain a database of local referral information. Practice secretaries and administrators are often a great source of this sort of knowledge and have a great deal of experience in how the local health services and referral systems work.
	It is also important to become familiar with the key national referral initiatives (e.g. the two-week wait) and local referral guidelines.

1.4c	**S Skills in managing the interface between primary and secondary care**

Our tips	The 'interface' refers to the various points of contact that occur between primary and secondary care. Managing this interface involves a number of skills. These include maintaining good continuity of care, ensuring effective communication between health professionals (to hand over, share and take back clinical responsibility), dealing appropriately with patient demand for access to services and managing unrealistic patient expectations.
	Maintaining a log of your referrals or carrying out an audit of your interactions with secondary care will help to identify aspects that work well and areas for improvement. Problems arising around the interface between primary and secondary care can often be the cause of adverse events (e.g. delayed referrals)[11] and these are often highly suitable incidents for a significant event analysis (SEA) (see 'The essential knowledge' – statement 3.2: *Patient Safety* for more info on SEA).

1.5 Making available to the patient the appropriate services within the healthcare system

What this involves

1.5a	**S Communication skills for counselling, teaching and treating patients and their carers**

Our tips	Communication skills are central to the discipline of general practice – after all, GPs spend most of their working day talking to people. Part of the role of a GP involves gaining a broad understanding of a patient's overall care and being able to communicate this to the patient and to colleagues.
	Theory: read up on the main consultation models (see 'The essential knowledge' – statement 2: *The General Practice Consultation* for an overview) and counselling models (e.g. neurolinguistic programming [NLP], problem solving, cognitive behavioural therapy [CBT]). Teaching skills are discussed in 'The essential knowledge' – statement 3.7: *Teaching, Mentoring and Clinical Supervision*).
	Practice: actor-based workshops, observing how other doctors consult, joint surgeries, videoing consultations, patient and 360° team feedback are some of the best ways to improve communication skills.

1.5b	**S Organisational skills for record keeping, information management, teamwork, running a practice and auditing the quality of care**

Our tips	These individual skills are covered in more detail in 'The essential knowledge' – statements 3.1–3.7: *Personal and Professional Responsibilities* and statements 4.1–4.2: *Management*.

Although it is no longer a compulsory part of GP certification, trainees would be well advised to do at least one full audit (two cycles) during their primary care training. Trainees should be encouraged to get involved in the practice's business and clinical organisational meetings as these offer valuable practical experience of the nuts and bolt of running a practice. Find out how your practice organises patient record summarising.

1.6 Acting as an advocate for the patient

What this involves

1.6a	**A Developing and maintaining a relationship, and a style of communication, that treats the patient as an equal and does not patronise the patient, and S skills in effective leadership, negotiation and compromise**

Our tips	Many GPs identify strongly with the role of patient advocate and some see one of their most important tasks as being to steer their patients successfully through the health system in order to obtain the best possible outcome.[12]

GPs fulfil a number of other important roles in the NHS; in particular they are responsible for the health of their local population and for managing the use of limited health resources. This means it is not always possible for a GP to act exclusively in the sole interest of one individual patient without disadvantaging another. Because of this, tensions can arise in the consultation and negotiation, and compromise is often called for. GPs must balance their role of patient advocate with their other responsibilities to the wider NHS while maintaining an effective and equitable relationship with their patients.

As well as relating to patients, this competency also applies to dealings with other professionals (e.g. colleagues, secondary care, primary-care organisations, etc). This can be a good topic to explore in a group learning activity. Practice managers can often pass on handy tips on how they deal with difficult GPs!

Competence 2 – person-centred care

Being 'person-centred' is a way of thinking and acting that considers the patient as a unique person in his or her own unique context, taking into account his or her preferences and expectations at every step in the consultation.[13] It is based on the concepts of autonomy, human rights, choice and social inclusion, and is now considered a fundamental part of good medical practice. In large part this approach has been driven by changes in Western society, culture and political values, but there is also a large body of evidence that a person-centred approach results in higher patient satisfaction and better health outcomes.[14]

2.1 Adopting a person-centred approach in dealing with patients and their problems in the context of the patients' circumstances

What this involves

2.1a	**K The basic scientific knowledge and understanding of the individual, together with his or her aims and expectations in life and K the development of a frame of reference to understand and deal with the family, community, social and cultural dimensions in a person's attitudes, values and beliefs**
Our tips	In addition to directly asking patients, other strategies for gaining an understanding of the individual patient include reviewing the patient's notes for the observations of colleagues, relevant social issues and previous decisions about care the patient has made, looking at the other family members that are registered with the practice, and discussion with other professionals involved in the patient's care.
	Knowing individuals will help you get to know your community. If you have a particular concentration of certain ethnic or religious groups in your area, consider asking a community representative to come to the practice or your learning group to discuss cultural and religious values and health beliefs.
	Narrative-based medicine (NBM) has recently gained increasing prominence in primary care.[15] NBM is concerned with how patients construct stories out of life events, which they may or may not relate to their health. Patient narratives can provide the GP with an individually tailored framework for approaching a patient's problems holistically, and can help to identify a patient's preferred management options. Narratives also offer a framework for addressing non-bio-psycho-social qualities of health and disease such as spiritual and moral issues, which may form part of people's illnesses but are not covered by traditional health and illness models.

2.1b	**S** Mastering patient illness and disease concepts, and **S** skills and attitudes to apply these in practice
Our tips	Helman's 'folk model of illness'[16] and the 'health belief model'[17] are easy to understand and attempt to explain patient views of health and disease, and their resultant behaviour. However, they have been criticised in the past as they make the assumption that patient decisions are always predominantly rational and fail to take into account the role emotions may play in patients' decisions about their illnesses. Other models of health and disease that have been developed include biomedical, psychosomatic, humanistic, existential and transpersonal models.[18]

2.2 To use the general practice consultation to bring about an effective doctor–patient relationship, always respecting the patient's autonomy

What this involves

2.2a	**S** Adopting a patient-centred consultation model that explores the patient's ideas, concerns and expectations, integrates the doctor's agenda, finds common ground and negotiates a mutual plan for the future, and **S** communicating findings in an understandable and comprehensible way, helping patients to reflect on their own concepts and finding common ground for further decision making
Our tips	The consultation is central to general practice. One of the most popular and easy-to-use consultation models is Roger Neighbour's five-checkpoint model from *The Inner Consultation*:[7]

Five consultation tasks are defined; at each step the GP thinks 'Where shall we make for next and how shall we get there?'

1. Connecting – establishing a rapport with the patient.
2. Summarising – using eliciting skills to discover the patient's ideas, concerns, expectations and summarising these back to the patient.
3. Handing over – agreeing the doctor's and patient's agendas then negotiating, influencing and gift-wrapping these.
4. Safety-netting – ensuring an appropriate contingency plan has been made.
5. Housekeeping – clearing away any psychological debris from the consultation to ensure it has no harmful effect on the next.

Sharing management decisions with the patient, including potential disagreements over how limited resources should be used, may raise tricky ethical and communication issues, which need to be resolved skilfully without damaging the doctor–patient relationship.

The concept of eliciting the patient's ideas, concerns and expectations at each consultation was first made popular in the mid-1980s by Pendleton and colleagues,[8] and has become an accepted tenet of patient-centred medicine.

Remember there are non-verbal methods of communicating information to patients. Alternative methods of conveying information are patient information leaflets (on paper or online, e.g. from www.patient.co.uk), and the use of graphs and charts to explain risks and probabilities (e.g. BMI charts or cardiovascular risk charts).

2.2b	**A** Making decisions that respect the patient's autonomy
Our tips	In Western society, patient autonomy has become the overriding ethical principle in most medical decisions although there are still some notable exceptions to this (e.g. in the areas of child protection and euthanasia).
	In general practice, respecting autonomy involves eliciting and taking into account the patient's ideas, concerns and expectations, and involving the patient at all steps of his or her care, including over how uncertainty is managed. Conveying information in a way that is understandable to the patient is key to achieving this – the principle of *informed* consent. A GP should also take steps to maximise the ability of the patient to comprehend the information required to make a decision – the principle of capacity to consent.
	Remember that autonomy also applies to the doctor – GPs have the right to refuse to act in a way that they perceive to be against the best interests of their patient, for example.

2.2c	**A** Being aware of subjectivity in the medical relationship, from both the patient's side (feelings, values and preferences) and from the doctor's side (self-awareness of values, attitudes and feelings)
Our tips	Keep a diary of consultations where you and the patient differed over your views on how to proceed. Why did this occur? How did you come to a decision? How could you have handled the situation differently? How did you balance the autonomy of the patient against the needs of the community and your professional duties as a GP?
	Remember you can't please all the people all the time, but you can learn how to handle difficult situations more effectively. You'll inevitably have easier medical relationships with some patients than others. Balint groups explore this area further.[19]

The website www.dipex.org contains a database of interviews with patients (and their families) discussing their real-life experiences of health and illness.

2.3 Communicating to set priorities and to act in partnership

What this involves

2.3a	**S The skills and A attitude to establish a partnership and to achieve a balance between emotional distance and proximity to the patient**
Our tips	The first part of the consultation usually involves establishing a rapport with a patient. It can be helpful to initially focus on the common ground that you share with the patient. If a patient is prepared to wait for an appointment to see you instead of consulting with another doctor in the practice, it usually means you have done this task successfully.
	Clear professional boundaries exist in the relationship between doctors and patients that must not be crossed (see the GMC's *Good Medical Practice*[1]) although, as with most ethical issues, grey areas exist. For example, consider how you would react if a patient gives you a box of chocolates at Christmas? Or writes you a personal cheque for £50 as a thank you? Or offers to donate £5000 to the practice? What would you do if a patient asks you out for a drink after work? What if you are a GP working in a remote community (e.g. a Scottish island or western Australia) and your only social contacts are also your patients – how would you manage your social life in that situation?

2.4 Providing long-term continuity of care and coordinated care management as determined by the needs of the patient

What this involves

2.4a	**K Understanding and mastering the three aspects of continuity: personal continuity; episodic continuity (making the appropriate medical information available for each patient contact); and continuity of care (24 hours a day and 365 days a year).**
Our tips	Patients nowadays have more options than ever before for choosing where they obtain their health care. Most out-of-hours care is provided by organisations outside the practice, and in working hours patients may decide to ring NHS Direct or attend a walk-in centre rather than to visit their GP. Patients may also choose to be referred to a secondary-care service outside their immediate locality.

Despite these changes, many GPs and patients continue to place great value on the continuity of a personal doctor–patient relationship. Personal continuity is increasingly difficult to provide as the healthcare system becomes more fragmented and complex, so new concepts of continuity are emerging.[20]

Episodic continuity is affected to a great extent by the effectiveness of the communication between health professionals and their organisations (such as quality of referral processes, correspondence and handovers). One of the goals of the NHS National Programme for IT, which incorporates the centralised electronic patient record, is to use technology to improve episodic continuity.

Consider ways in which your surgery can optimise these three types of continuity, particularly in challenging situations (e.g. terminal care). Carry out a significant event analysis of a situation where care was compromised by poor continuity. Focus on how it could have been improved.

2.4b	**S The ability to help the patient understand and achieve an appropriate work–life balance**
Our tips	Despite the partial introduction of the European Working Time Directive, workers in the UK work the longest hours in Europe. According to UNISON, one in six workers now work over 60 hours a week and, as the elderly population is rising, greater numbers of workers have additional caring responsibilities at home.[21]

As a result, many workers experience considerable time-pressures and GPs often see patients in whom work-related stress is a contributing factor to their illness. This is commonly an important factor to consider with patients suffering from mental health-related problems. It is important to remain person-centred, however, and recognise that what constitutes an appropriate work–life balance for one individual will vary from another and may change throughout that individual's lifetime. This will depend on the person's particular motivational needs, the nature of his or her work, and the other relevant factors in his or her life. This competency therefore requires both a person-centred and a holistic approach.

2.4c	**S** The ability to utilise disease registers and data-recording templates effectively for opportunistic and planned monitoring of problems to ensure continuity of care between different healthcare providers

Our tips

In order to make sure that practice disease registers and templates are accurate and comprehensive, it is crucial that all the members of the primary-care team learn how their practice systems work and can fill in the templates correctly!

Find out how to record patient data correctly in your practice (the data clerk or the GP in charge of the QoF may be able to help). It is also worth talking to colleagues or visiting other practices to find out alternative ways of recording patient data. Review your practice disease registers for a specific chronic disease (e.g. COPD) – how accurate is the register and what are the problems with ensuring it is both accurate and complete? If you are really up for a challenge, learn how to create your own patient data-recording template and design one that you feel your practice needs.

Competence 3 – specific problem-solving skills

There are various conceptual models of problem solving in general practice. One of the key early models, developed in this context by Marinker, is the hypothetico-deductive model.[22] This involves the GP formulating a hypothesis to explain the observed symptoms and signs. From the hypothesis, a number of predictions of further symptoms and signs are deduced that should be observable as a consequence of the hypothesis.

For example, imagine an otherwise well child presents with a history of right-sided earache and a mild fever for three days. From the history, the GP may formulate the hypothesis that the child is suffering from simple otitis media. The GP will predict that the ear drum will be red and inflamed, which, if confirmed on examination, will confirm the hypothesis and allow the GP to make a further prediction that the child's condition will settle over the next few days. If the child fails to improve as predicted, the original hypothesis must be rejected (a complication may have occurred or the original diagnosis may have been wrong), so the GP informs the parent that if the child does not improve as predicted they should return for another assessment.

3.1 Relating specific decision-making processes to the prevalence and incidence of illness in the community

What this involves

3.1a	**K** Knowledge of the prevalence and incidence of disease
Our tips	Prevalence (the proportion of individuals in a population having a disease) and incidence (the number of newly diagnosed cases during a specific time period) differ between primary care, which is a largely unselected population, and secondary care, which has been selected.
	Disease prevalence and incidence (particularly in terms of possible and probable diagnoses) also differ significantly from one community to another. For example, the health issues encountered in a practice in a deprived city centre can be fairly different from a practice in an affluent commuter suburb.
	Chapter 7, 'The essential knowledge', contains the common GP conditions described in the knowledge base of the curriculum.

3.1b	**K Knowledge of the practice community (age–sex distribution, prevalence of chronic diseases)**

Our tips How GPs apply the epidemiological knowledge gleaned from a medical textbook to their everyday practice will depend on their knowledge of the characteristics of their local community. For example, a GP working in an area with a large student population may expect to see a number of patients presenting with sexual and mental health problems, whereas a GP working in a practice with a predominantly elderly population may expect to see a greater amount of chronic disease.

Knowledge of the community also involves a whole host of other aspects, including genetic, social, psychological, economic, occupational, cultural, religious, educational, language and communication factors.

Established GPs at the practice will have a good idea of the practice community. Carrying out some searches on the practice population or reviewing the QoF chronic disease data (and comparing it with the national average) can give a good idea of the characteristics of the registered patients. A quirky (non-evidence-based) tip: take a trip to the local supermarket during a lunch break and have a good look round at the shoppers – they are often the same punters who most frequently visit the surgery!

Find out what specific groups of patients are associated with your practice population (nursing homes, schools, probation hostels, homeless people, drug or substance abuse). Are there any particular issues related to common occupational health issues in your practice area (e.g. mining or industry)?

3.1c	**S Skills to apply specific decision making (using tools such as clinical reasoning and decision rules)**

Our tips Start by locating some useful and valid guidelines and decision rules for the more common problems you encounter. For example, guidelines and decision-trees are available for assessing and managing hypertension, diabetes, high cholesterol, asthma, raised PSA, dyspepsia, change in bowel habit and contraception (to name a few). Look at the RCGP curriculum website (www.rcgp-curriculum.org.uk) for more resources.

Talk to colleagues about the guidelines, decision tools or risk calculators they find easy to apply in practice, but be sure to check their validity to your local population. Have a look at the cardiovascular risk charts in the back of the BNF. The British Hypertension Society offers downloadable cardiovascular disease (CVD) risk calculators and tables from its website (www.bhsoc.org) and the NHS Clinical Knowledge Summaries website (http://cks.library.nhs.uk) provides an up-to-date source of clinical knowledge to support decisions on primary-care management. The Ottawa Ankle Rules are helpful for deciding whether a patient with an ankle injury requires an X-ray.

Many practice record systems have built-in decision support software and include risk calculators and other tools.

3.2 Selectively gathering and interpreting information from history taking, physical examination and investigations, and applying it to an appropriate management plan in collaboration with the patient

What this involves

3.2a	**K Knowledge of relevant questions in the history and items in the physical examination relevant to the problem presented**
Our tips	Unlike a medical student's general clerking, a GP history and examination needs to accurately target the patient's problem, without being so narrow as to miss potentially important information and signs. Having a disease-based or systems-based approach to history taking and examination does not usually work well in primary care, where patients and their symptoms are unselected, and a problem-based approach is generally more effective.[23] This is rather different from the approach adopted in medical school and secondary care, so a transition needs to be made.

3.2b	**K Knowledge of the patient's relevant context, including family and social factors**
Our tips	Problem-solving in general practice is highly context specific. The skills required relate not only to the natural history of the problems themselves, but also to the context in which the problems are encountered, the personal characteristics of the patients, the doctors who manage them, and the available resources. Often, the only way you will find out about a patient's 'relevant context' is if you ask the patient. A social history can provide extremely pertinent information; for example, a diagnosis of plantar fasciitis may seem a trivial nuisance to a GP who spends most of the day sitting at his or her desk, but could mean a postman is unable to work for several months.
	It is equally important not to let your knowledge of the patient's family or social background prejudice your decisions and to respect the confidentiality of all the family members and any other patients who may live in the same household.

Some practice records systems have a handy 'household' function that enables you to pull up the records of other patients registered at the same address – this can be useful if a patient's story sounds familiar but you can't quite remember why!

3.2c	**K Knowledge of available investigations and treatment resources**

Our tips	This is more than learning about the theory of which tests or treatments you would arrange to investigate a certain condition – it is also about learning the practicalities of where to arrange them and how to carry them out.
	Find out which investigations and treatments your practice offers patients on site. This may include blood tests, warfarin monitoring, near-patient testing, ECGs, spirometry, audiometry, physiotherapy, podiatry, counselling and community dietician services. You may find your practice already has this information handily compiled in a handbook or locum folder; if not you may have to collate the information for your own use.
	Also, find out where patients need to go to get other investigations or treatments that the practice does not provide – how does this affect how frequently you order them?

3.2d	**S History taking and physical examination skills, and skills in interpreting data**

Our tips	Most new GPs will have acquired sound history-taking and examination skills during their earlier training. The challenge for trainees is to learn how to adapt these skills to everyday general practice. This is a complex process and involves bringing together a host of clinical skills that may have been learned in different departments over many years. It takes time and practice to get it right. Learning how to consult effectively in the time available (on average about 10 minutes) is one of the most challenging aspects of being a GP.
	The key investigations used in primary care are listed in the knowledge base contained in many of the curriculum statements. They are listed in Chapter 7, 'The essential knowledge'.

3.2e	**A A willingness to involve the patient in the management plan**
Our tips	There has been a clear shift over the past few decades away from a traditional paternalistic consulting style to a patient-centred care. This learning outcome is explored further in domain 2 – person-centred care and Chapter 7, 'The essential knowledge' – statement 2: *The General Practice Consultation.*

3.3 Adopting appropriate working principles (e.g. incremental investigation, using time as a tool) and tolerating uncertainty

What this involves

3.3a	**A Adopting skills and attitudes to demonstrate curiosity, diligence and caring**
Our tips	Of course it is even more important to use these characteristics in daily practice, rather than just being able to demonstrate that you can do so when you choose!

3.3b	**S Adopting stepwise procedures in medical decision making, using time as a diagnostic and therapeutic tool**
Our tips	'The art of medicine consists in amusing the patient while nature cures the disease' (Voltaire).
	GPs have the advantage over most hospital-based doctors of a long-term relationship with their patients. If a diagnosis is unclear, one option is to allow the passage of time to reveal whether the patient's symptoms and signs develop into a pattern that becomes recognisable as an illness. The other outcome, which happens very often, is that over time the symptoms will fade away and may never be explained.
	It is extremely important to consider patient safety when using time as a diagnostic tool – this concept is described as 'safety-netting' in Roger Neighbour's five-checkpoint consultation model.[7] Potentially serious diagnoses must be excluded in order to minimise any risk of harm to the patient from a delay in diagnosis, and patients should be made aware of the expected natural history of their symptoms and any significant variations in the expected pattern that they should report to a doctor.

3.3c	**A Understanding and acceptance of the inevitability of uncertainty in primary-care problem solving and development of strategies that demonstrate this**

Our tips	Marinker described GPs as tolerating uncertainty, exploring probability and marginalising danger. Hospital specialists, in contrast, work towards reducing uncertainty, exploring possibility and marginalising error.[22]
	A competent GP has the necessary attitudes, knowledge and skills to enable them to conduct an effective consultation with a patient, to make an accurate and objective estimation of the risks and to manage those risks appropriately – 'dealing with uncertainty'. The uncertainty a GP perceives should ideally be proportional to the objective risks that truly exist, although in reality the perception of uncertainty is affected by a number of other factors, including the GP's mental state and previous experiences.
	Keeping a reflective diary, to record the consultations where a particularly high degree of uncertainty is felt, will assist you to reflect on the reasons why uncertainty is perceived. Discussing these issues with a mentor or trainer can be a very useful way of identifying some strategies to manage uncertainty and equip you to deal more effectively with the uncertainties that will inevitably arise in the future.

3.4 To intervene urgently when necessary

What this involves

3.4a	**S Specific decision-making skills for emergency situations**

Our tips	The adult decision-making process generally involves six stages:

1. Defining the problem
2. Collecting information
3. Exploring the options
4. Drawing up a plan
5. Executing the plan
6. Reviewing the outcome.

In emergency situations, however, decision making is primarily a reactive process and there is insufficient time to go through the stages properly. As a result, it is easy to make bad decisions under pressure.

For this reason, the actions to be taken in an emergency situation should be carefully planned out beforehand so that as few decisions as possible need to be made at the time an emergency event occurs. Practically, this means familiarising yourself with your practice's emergency procedures and plans (e.g. fire, personal attack, flu pandemics) and regularly running through emergency clinical and resuscitation protocols and drills.

Decision making under pressure is a difficult skill to practice and it is not easy to predict how individuals will behave in emergency situations, which by their very nature are themselves unpredictable. Advanced Life Support (ALS), Advanced Trauma Life Support (ATLS) and other emergency management courses usually include simulations of emergencies to enable learners to practise these decision-making and leadership skills.[24]

3.4b	**S Specific skills in emergency procedures that may occur in primary-care situations**
Our tips	Fortunately, emergency procedures are needed relatively rarely in general practice. For this reason it can be very easy for these skills to get rusty so a strategy for ensuring you remain up to date is important.
	Basic Life Support (BLS) training for adults and children is recommended on a regular basis (at least every 1–2 years), not least because the protocols are frequently updated. If your practice has a defibrillator, you must find out how to use it and check it is properly maintained and serviced. Every practice should have an anaphylaxis kit, particularly when vaccinations are given, and this must also be checked regularly to ensure the drugs and equipment don't go out of date (adrenaline has a relatively short shelf-life).
	All GP trainees should make arrangements to obtain sufficient out-of-hours experience during their training. The other specific emergency skills will depend on individual practice factors, such as the location of the practice (remote practices tend to experience more dramatic emergencies than practices near to A&E departments) and the characteristics of the local population. Carrying out critical event analyses and team skills assessments will help identify what training the practice team requires.

3.5 Managing conditions that may present early and in an undifferentiated way

What this involves

3.5a	**K Knowledge of when to wait and reassure, and when to initiate additional diagnostic and therapeutic action**
Our tips	This involves knowing when it is appropriate to wait and see, when to refer, when to arrange a follow-up appointment or carry out some investigations to exclude potentially serious diseases. An accurate estimation of risk allows a GP to use their feelings of uncertainty to make an appropriate management plan and to successfully share this uncertainty with the patient.
	GPs must learn about the principle of 'red flags'; these are specific symptoms and signs that indicate further action is required. Red flags exist for a range of common symptoms seen in primary care, including back pain, dyspepsia and headache.
	The National Library for Health (www.library.nhs.uk) has a guidelines finder with over 2000 guidelines available. The National Institute for Health and Clinical Excellence (NICE) has produced referral guidelines for GPs on managing patients with suspected cancer, available on its website: www.nice.org.uk.

3.6 Making effective and efficient use of diagnostic and therapeutic interventions

What this involves

3.6a	**K Knowledge that symptoms and signs vary in their predictive value, as do findings from ancillary tests**
Our tips	Predictive value is a fundamental statistical concept. The predictive value of a finding or a test varies with the prevalence (i.e. the pre-test probability) of the disease. This is particularly relevant to primary care where the population has a lower prevalence of serious disease than in secondary care. Generally, the rarer the disease in a population, the lower the positive predictive value of a finding or test.
	This is in contrast with the sensitivity or specificity of a finding or a test, which relates to the test itself and does not depend on the prevalence of the disease.

Look into the predictive values (both positive and negative) of a few commonly used tests. For example: D-dimers in suspected deep-vein thrombosis, anti-endomysial antibodies in coeliac disease and troponins in the diagnosis of chest pain. How does knowledge of the predictive value of a particular test help with the management of an individual patient?

The Applied Knowledge Test (AKT) component of the new MRCGP tests knowledge of basic statistics. Candidates should learn the definitions and concepts of the common terms used in evidence-based medicine (EBM) (see condensed statement 3.5 in Chapter 7, 'The essential knowledge', for a handy checklist).

3.6b	**K An understanding of the cost-efficiency and cost–benefit of tests and treatments**
Our tips	In health care, cost-efficiency is a measure of the total healthcare spending for a service (or group of services associated with a specific patient population) compared against a clinical outcome over a specified time period. A cost–benefit analysis is used for determining which alternative intervention is likely to provide the greatest health improvement for a proposed amount of investment.

Competence 4 – a comprehensive approach

An effective GP must be able to manage the multiple complaints and co-morbidities of their patients. When a patient seeks medical advice, he or she has become ill as a person and may not be able to differentiate between the effects of his or her various conditions. The challenge of addressing multiple health issues simultaneously requires GPs to develop the skills needed to both interpret the issues and to prioritise them in partnership with the patient. GPs also provide rehabilitation for their patients and, in the end phase of a patient's life, palliative care. A GP must be able to coordinate the care provided by other healthcare professionals and agencies.

4.1 To simultaneously manage multiple complaints and pathologies, both acute and chronic health problems

What this involves

4.1a	**K An understanding of the concept of co-morbidity in a patient and the S skill to manage the concurrent health problems experienced by a patient through identification, exploration, negotiation, acceptance and prioritisation**
Our tips	Co-morbidity describes the effects of any additional diseases of an individual patient other than the disease primarily being considered. It is particularly relevant in the care of the elderly and also increasingly a matter of concern in patients suffering from mental health problems who often have neglected physical health problems.
	Keep a record of a handful of patients you see with four or more active problems – then review their notes and medications, and consider how these problems may interact, both physically and in psycho-social ways.
4.1b	**S Skill in using the medical record and other information**
Our tips	Early on in your training have a tutorial on how to use your practice computer system. It is not uncommon for modern GP trainees to pick up these skills fairly quickly and become more adept at using the computer system than some of the more experienced GPs in the practice!

4.1c	**S The skill to seek, and the A attitude to use the best evidence in practice**
Our tips	In this outcome, the *attitude* is about wanting to practice evidence-based medicine (EBM) on a regular basis.
	The two main aspects to this *skill* are being able to interpret the evidence, so as to have an answer to your question, and then being able to apply it in practice. This involves knowing where to look and learning how to ask the right question. Good places to look for high-quality evidence include the Cochrane Library, Clinical Evidence, Best Evidence and in original journals (two journals particularly relevant to general practice are the *British Journal of General Practice* and the *British Medical Journal*).
	Also, try the primary-care question answering service from the NHS National Electronic Library for Health (www.library.nhs.uk) – asking a good question is crucial to finding the information you are looking for (look up the PICO format by going to www.cebm.net and following the link to 'questions' under 'doing EBM').
	Using the best evidence requires the development of sound EBM skills. *The Centre for Evidence-Based Medicine* (www.cebm.net) provides a number of resources to help with the development of EBM skills. Many training practices have a journal club where EBM skills can be practised.

4.2 To promote health and wellbeing by applying health promotion and disease prevention strategies appropriately

What this involves

4.2a	**S The ability to understand the concept of health**
Our tips	The World Health Organization defines health as 'a state of complete physical, mental and social well-being and not merely the absence of disease or infirmity'.[25] This definition highlights how health should be considered holistically, rather than just focusing on physical health.

4.2b	**S The ability to promote health on an individual basis as part of the consultation**
Our tips	There are numerous health promotion opportunities in a consultation. A few common examples include smoking cessation, diet and exercise advice, sexual health screening, and cervical smears. The skill comes in tailoring the messages you want to give to the individual patient and framing them in a way the patient will be able to assimilate.

4.2c	**S** The ability to promote health through a health promotion or disease prevention programme within the primary-care setting and **K** understanding the role of the GP in health promotion activities to the community
Our tips	This outcome is covered in Chapter 7, 'The essential knowledge' – statement 5: *Healthy People*.

4.2d	**S** Understanding and recognising the importance of ethical tensions between the needs of the individual and the community, and acting appropriately
Our tips	Keep a log of any resource dilemmas that arise in your practice, and discuss them with your trainer or learning group. What are the basic ethical principles involved and how can you address the dilemma?
	Consider the concept of 'opportunity cost' in health care – this is the cost paid, both economically and in terms of people's wellbeing, when we give up something in order to get something else.

4.3 To manage and coordinate health promotion, prevention, cure, care, rehabilitation and palliation

What this involves

4.3a	**K** Understanding the complex nature of health problems in general practice and **K** understanding the variety of possible approaches and **S** the ability to use different approaches for an individual patient and to modify these according to an individual's need
Our tips	GPs are concerned with the health of entire families as well as individuals. Not all patients are the same so a successful GP needs a repertoire of skills and to be able to select which to use with which patient. Patients can be young, old, well, ill, poorly informed or well informed, anxious or laidback and from many different cultures and nationalities.
	There are inter-patient and inter-doctor variations. Try sitting in with different doctors to observe some of this variety. You will observe some GPs seem particularly adept at communicating with particular types of patients. If there are only a few GPs at your practice, consider arranging a swap with a colleague at another practice.
	In addition to a portfolio of skills used during the conventional office-based consultations, think about skills needed for alternative consultations (e.g. drop-in services, home visits, telephone or email consultations, internet advice, etc.).

4.3b	**S** To coordinate teamwork in primary care

Our tips	There is lots of theory written about teamwork. Relevant models for general practice include:

- Myers–Briggs personality profiles[26]
- Belbin's team roles[27]
- Bruce Tuckman's group development model[28]
- Maslow's motivational needs hierarchy model[29]
- Leadership styles.

The website www.businessballs.com contains information on these models of team theory and leadership, and offers some games and exercises to encourage team-building. A GP's role includes coordinating and leading a team – observe and evaluate others doing it and talk to your trainer or practice manager about creating opportunities for you to try out being a team leader on a practice project. Remember to ask for and record constructive feedback.

Competence 5 – community orientation

GPs, as family and community doctors, have a responsibility that stretches beyond the boundaries of a consultation with an individual patient. The work of a GP is determined by the make-up of his or her community and therefore GPs must understand the characteristics of the community in which they work, including socio-economic and health features. Healthcare systems are rationed in some form in all societies, and GPs have a clinical, ethical and moral duty to influence health policy in their community.

5.1 To reconcile the health needs of individual patients and the health needs of the community in which they live, balancing these with available resources

What this involves

5.1a	**K An understanding of the health needs of communities through the epidemiological characteristics of their populations and K an understanding of the impact of poverty, ethnicity and local epidemiology on a local community's health**
Our tips	To provide effective services, the local GPs, the practices and the local NHS must tailor their services to the particular needs of the community (see 3.1b).

5.1b	**K An understanding of the interrelationships between health and social care**
Our tips	In the past, the various agencies involved in health and social care have not always succeeded in coordinating their responses to patient needs. This has led to people being assessed repeatedly and valuable information being lost. People often complain that they are not kept informed about what is happening with their health care.
	Find out about the Single Assessment Process (SAP) that was introduced following the National Service Framework for Older People in 2001.[30] A key principle is that there is a single person-centred and holistic assessment to which the various health and social services contribute.

5.1c	**K To be aware of inequalities in healthcare provision**

Our tips	Have you heard the phrase 'postcode lottery' in the media?

Thirty years ago a GP called Julian Tudor Hart first proposed 'the inverse care law'.[31] This describes how socio-economically deprived people, who need health care the most, are the least likely to get it. In contrast, those with less need for health care tend to use the health services more effectively.

The King's Fund provides reports on the impact of inequalities in healthcare provision (www.kingsfund.org.uk).

5.1d	**K An understanding of the structure of the healthcare system and its economic limitations**

Our tips	The National Institute for Health and Clinical Excellence (www.nice.org.uk) is an independent organisation responsible for providing national guidance on the promotion of good health and the prevention and treatment of ill health. This process includes appraising treatments for cost-effectiveness and recommending treatments for the NHS.

5.1e	**K An understanding of the roles of the other professionals involved in community policy relating to health**

Our tips	On a community level, the local PCT is responsible for public health and employing local public health specialists.

The Faculty of Public Health (www.fphm.org.uk) is a faculty of the Royal College of Physicians and the standard-setting body for specialists in public health. The Health Protection Agency (www.hpa.org.uk) is an independent body that protects the health and wellbeing of the population.

The Public Health Resource Unit (www.phru.nhs.uk) supports people and NHS organisations in their public health role and provides information and educational resources.

5.1f	**K An understanding of the importance of practice- and community-based information in the quality assurance of each doctor's practice**

Our tips	The Quality and Outcomes Framework (QoF) was introduced as part of the GP contract in 2004. It is an annual incentive scheme that awards practices financially for hitting targets in the following areas:

- Managing some of the common chronic diseases, e.g. asthma, diabetes, epilepsy, hypertension, hypothyroidism
- How well the practice is organised
- How patients rate their experience at the practice (recorded by a patient survey).

The QoF gives an indication of the overall achievement of a surgery. Practices that deliver high-quality care across a range of areas score points that are translated into money ('points mean prizes'). The higher the points scored, the higher the financial reward for the practice. The payment is adjusted to take account of surgery workload by adjusting the value of the points to reflect the relative health of patients in the local community.

Although controversial, there is no doubt that the introduction of the QoF has had a big impact on the everyday work of GP practices. Speak to your practice manager or the GP leading on the QoF to find out some of the pros and cons.

QoF results for practices can be viewed at www.qof.ic.nhs.uk. You can find information on the patient surveys at www.gp-patient.co.uk.

5.1g	**K An understanding of how healthcare systems can be used by the patient and the doctor (referral procedures, co-payments, sick leave, legal issues, etc.) in their own context**

Our tips	People do not only use the healthcare system to obtain health care. Many people visit their GP with a different agenda. Here are some of the more common non-medical agendas:

- To be referred to a specialist (for various non-medical reasons)
- To obtain a sickness certificate
- To get their passport application signed
- To request a letter or medical report
- To attend for a medical examination (e.g. for life insurance).

Arrange a tutorial on the sickness certification system (in particular Med 3, 4 and 5) and medical reports for claiming Incapacity Benefit and Disability Living Allowance.

5.1h	**S The ability to reconcile the needs of the individual with the needs of the community in which they live**
Our tips	Part of the traditional GP role was that of 'gatekeeper'. The idea of GPs rationing access to health care is politically sensitive in the current era of patient choice, and although much of this task has been shifted to referral management centres and PCTs, it remains an implicit part of a modern GP's role.
	A key aspect of the community-orientated nature of general practice is the role that GPs play in the rationing of healthcare resources and the influencing on health policy in the community; the NHS has finite resources and a significant proportion of NHS spending happens in primary care. GPs need to be able to balance the needs of individual patients against the needs of the whole community they serve.
	The Public Health Resource Unit (www.phru.nhs.uk) produces a number of board games and other educational resources on commissioning and allocating health resources, designed for use by learning groups.

5.1i	**K An understanding of GPs' role in the commissioning of health care**
Our tips	GPs are taking an increasing role in the commissioning of local healthcare services. Practice-based commissioning (PBC) is a recent government policy intended to encourage practices and other primary-care professionals to become involved in the commissioning of services. Through PBC, it is hoped that clinicians on the front line will be able to become more involved in commissioning decisions.
	Many practices are grouping together to form local consortia and other organisations for the purposes of delivering PBC – this may involve commissioning and designing new services tailored for the local community.

Competence 6 – a holistic approach

Holism in general practice involves the integration of the physical, psychological and social components of health problems, and is well established as being central to good consulting practice.

6.1 To use bio-psycho-social models, taking into account cultural and existential dimensions

What this involves

6.1a	**K** Knowledge of the holistic concept and implications for the patients' care
Our tips	Kemper defines holism as 'caring for the whole person in the context of the person's values, their family beliefs, their family system and their culture in the larger community, and considering a range of therapies based on the evidence of their benefits and cost'.[32] It can also be described as the integration of physical, psychological and social components of health problems in making diagnoses and planning management.
	The concept of holism and the key references are summarised very well in the core curriculum statement *Being a General Practitioner.*

6.1b	**S** The ability to understand a patient as a bio-psycho-social whole
Our tips	… a patient is also a person too!
	The RCGP's triaxial model (biological, psychological and social) forms a basic framework for a GP to consider a patient holistically, including physical, emotional, family, social and environmental circumstances.[33]
	Cultural and existential issues (those relating to people's experience of existence) are also considered part of holism but are not explicitly covered by the triaxial model.

6.1c	**S** The skills to transform holistic understanding into practical measures
Our tips	This is about translating theory into practice. This can be assessed by videoing your consultations and reviewing them with a trainer or mentor, considering the various aspects of holistic care. Role-play with colleagues or actors briefed to include holistic aspects in the consultation can also help you to practise these skills.

6.1d	**K Knowledge of the cultural background and beliefs of the patient, in so far as they are relevant to healthcare, and A tolerance and understanding towards patients' experiences, beliefs, values and expectations as they affect healthcare delivery**

Our tips

This is partly about having an awareness of the cultural aspects relevant to particular groups of patients you may see, and partly about gaining specific knowledge of individual patient's beliefs. For example, you may be at a loss to explain why a patient seems reluctant to take the lansoprazole capsules you have prescribed for their heartburn, until you discover the capsules contain gelatin, which is an animal product that the patient is unwilling to consume for religious reasons.

Tolerance does not mean treating everyone exactly the same but involves recognising and respecting an individual's beliefs and cultural practices. Making unwarranted assumptions about a patient's beliefs can result in you putting your foot in it and appearing very foolish. Few people are reluctant to discuss their culture or beliefs yet many GPs worry excessively about causing offence if they ask about them – it is better to plead ignorance rather than make assumptions!

Identify a specific situation in which you have struggled with being tolerant and understanding towards a patient. This can be a sensitive subject, so you may prefer to reflect on this alone, or preferably discuss it with a trainer or trusted colleague – try to identify what happened, then why the difficulties arose, and come up with some alternative ways of dealing with the situation.

The three essential application features

The essential application features described in the curriculum are the important factors that are always present in the background of a consultation and exert a strong effect on how a GP's knowledge and skills are applied in everyday general practice.

1. Contextual aspects of care

This includes an awareness of the environment in which a GP practices, the working conditions, the community, local culture, financial and regulatory frameworks and guidelines; the impact of workload and the practice facilities; the particular context of the individual patient and his or her family and background.

2. Attitudinal aspects of care

This requires a GP to be aware of his or her own attitudes and capabilities; the ability to identify ethical aspects of clinical practice and to understand his or her personal ethics and values; achieving a good balance between work and private life.

3. Scientific aspects of care

This involves the GP adopting a critical and evidence-based approach to daily practice and maintaining this through continuing learning, professional development and quality improvement.

Essential feature 1 – contextual aspects

This involves an understanding of the context of general practice and the environment in which GPs work, including the local working conditions, community, culture, financial and regulatory frameworks and guidelines; the impact of workload and the practice facilities; the particular context of the individual patient and his or her family and background.

EF 1.1	**The impact of the local community (including socio-economic and workplace factors, geography and culture) on patient care**
Our tips	'No man is an island …'[34] Reflect on the features of your practice's local community that particularly influence the delivery of patient care – how does the community exert this influence and are there any factors that you can modify? Consider how this contrasts with other practices; practices may be located in inner-city or rural communities, in affluent or deprived areas, and so on.

EF 1.2	**The impact of overall workload on the care given to the individual patient and the facilities (e.g. staff, equipment) available to deliver that care**
Our tips	What length appointments does your practice offer patients and why? Do all the GPs offer the same-length consultations? Look up the evidence around consultations times and quality of care. Consider the factors that stress your practice's ability to deliver care (demand for appointments, staff holidays, unexpected sick leave, etc.) and the plans in place to address these, as well as the practice-based factors that link to high-quality care.

EF 1.3	**The financial and legal frameworks in which health care is given at a practice level**
Our tips	This includes being familiar with relevant aspects of common law, employment law, important acts of Parliament and professional guidelines for best practice. It also involves gaining an understanding of how general practices are financed and the various types of GP contract. Speak to the senior partner or the practice manager about how these various frameworks are implemented and managed in your practice.

EF 1.4	**The impact of the doctor's personal housing and working environment on the care that he or she provides**
Our tips	This is how one of the authors justified buying themselves a new kitchen! Consider how the fabric of the building you work in affects the care you offer patients. This includes the number of available consulting and treatment rooms, the size and comfort of the waiting rooms (e.g. do you have easily accessible chairs for infirm patients?) and the equipment you have in the practice (e.g. is there an ECG machine and a spirometer or do you have to persuade patients to attend the local hospital or diagnostic centre for these investigations?).

Essential feature 2 – attitudinal aspects

This requires the GP to be aware of his or her own attitudes and capabilities; the ability to identify ethical aspects of clinical practice and to understand his or her personal ethics and values; achieving a good balance between work and private life.

EF 2.1	**Your own professional capabilities and values**
Our tips	Reflective practice is an essential skill in modern professional practice, and a significant aspect of this involves gaining an understanding of your own values. You can also assess your capabilities objectively (e.g. through the use of rating scales and assessments) and from feedback from others.
	The Johari window* is a useful conceptual tool for assessing and improving your self-awareness. You can find it on the Businessballs website (www.businessballs.com).
	*Interestingly, Luft and Ingham created the name 'Johari' in the 1960s by combining their first names, Joe and Harry.[35]

EF 2.2	**Ethical aspects of clinical practice (including prevention, diagnostics, therapy, factors that influence lifestyle)**
Our tips	The four basic ethical principles of autonomy, beneficence, non-maleficence and justice are a good foundation for making ethical judgements. Become alert to the classic ethical dilemmas of general practice – some are fairly obvious arenas for ethical debates in the new MRCGP Clinical Skills Assessment (CSA) such as abortion, chaperones, confidentiality, euthanasia, genetic testing, informed consent, rationing of health care and whistle-blowing. A learning group is an ideal forum for discussing cases that raise complex ethical issues as it encourages members to form their own opinions and exposes people to alternative ideas and perspectives.
	Less obvious ethical issues crop up all the time in day-to-day practice. For example, considering to what extent to twist someone's arm when attempting to persuade them to stop engaging in what you believe to be a harmful activity, such as smoking, involves a judgement based on the conflicting principles of autonomy and beneficence.

EF 2.3	**Understanding self – this is about understanding that your attitudes and feelings are important determinants of how you practice**
Our tips	'*Know yourself*' was inscribed at the entrance to the Temple of Apollo at Delphi – Apollo was considered to be an ancient god of healing.
	A reflective diary can help to identify situations in which your attitudes and feelings influenced your practice. This should include both positive and negative experiences.
	Psychological concepts such as transference (the patient unconsciously transferring feelings arising from another relationship to the GP) and counter-transference (the GP experiencing feelings through identification with the emotions, experiences or problems of the patient) can provide some useful insights. Consider how these phenomena may affect your consultations (especially if a patient makes you feel particularly angry, upset or anxious but you aren't sure why).

EF 2.4	**Justifying and clarifying personal ethics**
Our tips	A person's espoused values and their real-life behaviour can often differ (hence the need for a criminal justice system). It's worth spending time to thrash out your thoughts on some of the common ethical issues that are bound to come up as a working GP. Then, when you meet these situations, you will have an opportunity to reflect and further develop your personal ethics. If you don't take time to reflect on your actions when ethical issues arise in practice, you may not be aware if your behaviour starts to deviate from the values you support.
	See 'The essential knowledge' – statement 3.3: *Clinical Ethics and Values-Based Practice.*

EF 2.5	**The interaction between work and your private life; striving for a good balance between them**
Our tips	Work–life balance is important for GPs as well as their patients. A good balance will depend on your personal circumstances and personality although every GP should be aware of the phenomenon of 'burnout' and ways to prevent it. Burnout is a syndrome of emotional exhaustion, depersonalisation, low productivity and low achievement. It is a particular problem in the medical profession.[36]
	The RCGP produces a useful leaflet *Stress and General Practice*, which can be downloaded from its website: www.rcgp.org.uk/pdf/ISS_INFO_22_FEB05.pdf.

Essential feature 3 – scientific aspects

This involves the GP adopting a critical and evidence-based approach to daily practice and maintaining this through continuing learning, professional development and quality improvement.

EF 3.1	**Familiarity with the general principles, methods and concepts of scientific research and the fundamentals of statistics**
Our tips	This learning outcome is covered in 'The essential knowledge' – statement 3.6: *Research and Academic Activity.*

EF 3.2	**Having a thorough knowledge of: the scientific backgrounds of pathology, symptoms and diagnosis, therapy and prognosis, epidemiology, decision theory, theories about the forming of hypotheses and problem solving, and preventive health care**
Our tips	This is clearly a huge area and most of the detail here is covered in Chapter 7, 'The essential knowledge'. However, you may need to look outside the curriculum to find the scientific and theoretical background to decision theory, hypothesis forming and problem solving.

EF 3.3	**Critical reading of medical literature and putting the literature into practice**
Our tips	There are several good resources, including websites and books, on critical appraisal. Look at the RCGP curriculum resources website for some of these: www.rcgp-curriculum.org.uk.

Also consider:

- Does your practice have a journal club?
- If so, how do you identify which papers to read?
- Do you know how to find high-quality papers that answer your (well-framed) clinical questions? Look at: www.cebm.net
- Some adopt a 'scan the key journals' approach, whereas others focus on articles based on clinical interest (what are the benefits and risks of these approaches?)
- Try out the 'Journal Watch' services offered by some publications and websites such as the RCGP (www.rcgp.org.uk/library_/library_home/journal_watch.aspx), Doctors.net (www.doctors.net.uk) and Global Family Doctor (www.globalfamilydoctor.com)

- Hot-topics courses are popular and are an efficient way to keep your awareness of recent developments up to date, although you are relying on other people to set the agenda.

EF 3.4	**Developing and maintaining continuing learning and quality improvement**

Our tips	All working GPs and doctors in training should maintain a learning portfolio including a personal development plan. Both GP trainees (in primary care) and established GPs are required to undergo annual appraisals, and regular revalidation is shortly to be introduced. The NHS appraisals toolkit has some useful tools for this and is becoming increasingly popular among GPs: www.appraisals.nhs.uk.
	Read Chapter 3, 'Learning the curriculum', for more information on identifying your learning needs and on continuing professional development.
	Quality improvement involves not only personal development but also improving the service offered by the whole practice. Find out if your practice has a practice development plan and look at the RCGP website (www.rcgp.org.uk) for more information on practice quality improvement.

Psychomotor skills and the knowledge base

The key practical and clinical skills and items of knowledge described in the core curriculum statement and all the other statements have been summarised in the following chapter, 'The essential knowledge'.

References

1 General Medical Council. *Good Medical Practice* London: General Medical Council, 2006 (available at: www.gmc-uk.org [accessed June 2007]).

2 Royal College of General Practitioners/General Practitioners Committee. *Good Medical Practice for General Practitioners* London: RCGP, 2002.

3 *The European Definition of General Practice/Family Medicine* Barcelona: WONCA Europe, 2002.

4 Eve R. Meeting educational needs in general practice – learning with PUNs and DENs *Education for General Practice* 2000; **11**: 73–9.

5 Luft J and Ingham H. *The Johari Window: a graphic model of interpersonal awareness. Proceedings of the western training laboratory in group development* Los Angeles: UCLA, 1955.

6 Wilson A and Childs S. The relationship between consultation length, process and outcomes in general practice: a systematic review *British Journal of General Practice* 2002; **52**: 1012–20.

7 Neighbour R. *The Inner Consultation* Lancaster: MTP Press, 1987.

8 Pendleton D, Schofield T, Tate P, Havelock P. *The Consultation: an approach to teaching and learning* Oxford: Oxford Medical Publications, 1984.

9 www.primarycarecontracting.nhs.uk [accessed June 2007].

10 Campbell H, Hotchkiss R, Bradshaw N, Porteous M. Integrated care pathways *British Medical Journal* 1998; **316(7125)**: 133–7.

11 RCGP curriculum statement 3.2: *Patient Safety* London: RCGP, 2007.

12 Rees Jones I, Doyle L, Berney L, Kelly M. *Decision-Making in Primary Care: patients as partners in resource allocation* London: St George's Medical School, 2003.

13 Stewart M (ed.). *Patient-Centered Medicine: transforming the clinical method* Thousand Oaks, CA: Sage, 1995.

14 Kinnersley P, Stott N, Peters TJ, Harvey I. The patient-centredness of consultations and outcome in primary care *British Journal of General Practice* 1999; **49(446)**: 711–16.

15 Greenhalgh T and Hurwitz B (eds). *Narrative Based Medicine* London: BMJ Books, 1998.

16 Helman C G. Disease versus illness in general practice *Journal of the Royal College of General Practitioners* 1981; **31**: 548–62.

17   Rosenstock I. *Historical Origins of the Health Belief Model*. Health Education Monographs Vol. 2, No. 4, 1974.

18   Tamm ME. Models of health and disease *British Journal of Medical Psychology* 1993; **66**: 213–28.

19   Balint M. *The Doctor, His Patient and the Illness* London: Pitman Medical Publishing, 1964.

20   Freeman G and Hjortdahl P. What future for continuity of care in general practice? *British Medical Journal* 1997; **314**: 1870–3.

21   www.unison.org.uk [accessed June 2007].

22   Marinker M and Peckham M (eds). *Clinical Futures* London: BMJ Books, 1998.

23   Deighan M. *RCGP Curriculum for General Practice – learning and teaching guide* London: RCGP, 2006.

24   www.resus.org.uk [accessed June 2007].

25   *Constitution of the World Health Organization* Geneva: WHO, 1946.

26   Briggs Myers I. *Manual: the Myers–Briggs Type Indicator* Palo Alto, CA: CPP, 1962.

27   Belbin RM. *Management Teams. Why they succeed or fail* London: Butterworth-Heinemann, 1981 (www.belbin.com [accessed June 2007]).

28   Tuckman BW. Developmental sequence in small groups *Psychology Bulletin* 1965; **63**: 384–99.

29   Maslow A. *Motivation and Personality* New York: Harper, 1970.

30   Department of Health. *National Service Framework for Older People* London: Department of Health, 2001 (available at: www.dh.gov.uk).

31   Tudor Hart J. The inverse care law *Lancet* 1971; **i**: 405–12.

32   Kemper KJ. Holistic pediatrics = good medicine *Pediatrics* 2000; **105**: 214–18.

33   Working Party of the Royal College of General Practitioners, 1972.

34   John Donne (1572–1631).

35   Luft J and Ingham H. *Of Human Interaction* Palo Alto: National Press, 1969.

36   Kirwan M and Armstrong D. Investigation of burnout in a sample of British general practitioners *British Journal of General Practice* 1995; **45**: 259–60.

7 The essential knowledge

The condensed statements

This section of the book contains the core knowledge and skills of general practice described in the 32 statements of the RCGP Curriculum for Specialty Training for General Practice. For each statement, we have extracted the key educational content and packaged it into four easy-to-understand sections, as described in Table 7.1.

Table 7.1

Sections within each condensed statement	
The condensed knowledge	This contains the core items of knowledge contained in the statement's knowledge base (not all statements have this section)
The condensed skills	This contains the key skills described in the statement and our interpretation of how they apply to the topic or group of patients concerned
The condensed know-how	This contains the key applied knowledge extracted from the learning outcomes for the statement
The condensed resources	This contains a selection of useful educational resources for learning and teaching the statement

Our tips for learning and teaching

Throughout this chapter we have included a variety of useful tips and specific resources to help support the learning and teaching of each statement. Some of these are taken from the resources listed in the full curriculum statements and others are derived from other sources including the published literature and the advice of established trainers, course organisers and GP educationalists.

To the right-hand side of each description of knowledge or skill we have included a box for you tick or score. This depends on how you plan to use the book in your learning process.

Table 7.2

Tick or score	
Tick ☑	You can use the condensed curriculum as a checklist, ticking each box when you have read the item concerned, or marking that you are confident that you have mastered the relevant item of knowledge, skill or know-how
Score	You can use 'The essential knowledge' as a *self-assessment confidence rating scale* by giving each piece of knowledge, skill or know-how a score from **1–5**:
	1 – I am not at all confident in this area of knowledge or ability **2** – I have some knowledge or ability here, but don't feel I am competent **3** – I am probably competent at this but would like to learn more **4** – I feel confident my current knowledge or ability is competent **5** – I am simply awesome at this!
	This process can help you identify the knowledge and skills you feel least confident about and assist in setting priorities for planning your learning. First, focus on addressing the items that you scored '**1**', then move on to those marked '**2**' and so on.
	It is advisable to ask a trainer or mentor who has observed your performance to review your scores in order to check that your subjective assessment is a true reflection of your abilities. If there is more than one point of disagreement between you and your trainer over a particular item or knowledge or skill, reflect on why this might be.
	An electronic version of this confidence rating scale is available at: www.rcgp-curriculum.org.uk

Index of condensed statements

Statement 1: *Being a General Practitioner*

The first curriculum statement, *Being a General Practitioner*, describes the six core competences and three essential features of general practice that form the template on which all the other curriculum statements are based.

The six domains of core competence are:

1. Primary care management

2. Person-centred care

3. Specific problem-solving skills

4. A comprehensive approach

5. Community orientation

6. A holistic approach.

The three essential application features are:

1. **Contextual** – using the context of the person, the family, the community and their culture

2. **Attitudinal** – basing actions on the doctor's professional capabilities, values and ethics

3. **Scientific** – adopting a critical and research-based approach to practice and maintaining this through continuing learning and quality improvement.

The core competences and essential application features are explored in detail in Chapter 6, 'The core competences'.

The condensed resources

There are numerous web-based educational resources available to GP trainees, trainers and established GPs that support learning and teaching across the breadth of general practice. We have identified a handful of resources that offer a wide range of material relevant to large areas of the curriculum. To avoid repeating these resources in every condensed statement, they are listed here as wide-ranging curriculum resources.

The RCGP curriculum website: www.rcgp-curriculum.org.uk

Provides a wealth of information on the curriculum, GP training and education, including the online curriculum map and a database of educational and training resources that have been specially selected to support the learning and teaching of the curriculum. Also has information on the nMRCGP assessments, and news on educational courses and events. The RCGP website also enables college members and associates in training to gain free access to a range of popular subscription-only journals including:

- BMJ (*British Medical Journal*)
- BJGP (*British Journal of General Practice*)
- *Education for Primary Care*
- *Evidence-Based Medicine*
- JAMA (*Journal of the American Medical Association*)
- *Journal of Epidemiology and Community Health*
- *The Lancet*
- *Medical Education*
- *Work Based Learning in Primary Care*.

Clinical Knowledge Summaries: http://cks.library.nhs.uk

Provides updated evidence-based summaries of clinical knowledge aimed to support health professionals working in primary care, incorporating PRODIGY guidance.

Doctors.net: www.doctors.net.uk

Offers a range of educational resources for doctors, including online textbooks and databases, a Journal Watch service and a wide range of accredited learning modules on important general practice topics.

GPNotebook: www.gpnotebook.co.uk

A popular and accessible online encyclopaedia of medicine that is a particularly useful resource for learning the knowledge base contained within the curriculum. It also offers GP Notebook Educational Modules ('GEMS'), which allow learners to test themselves on important GP topics.

The National Library for Health: www.library.nhs.uk

Contains numerous resources of interest to GP learners and teachers, including key sources of evidence (Bandolier, Clinical Knowledge Summaries, Cochrane Library), a guidelines finder, NICE Guidance, NLH Protocols & Care Pathways, books, journals and bibliographical databases, image banks, patient resources (DIPEX, NHS Direct Online, Patient.co.uk) and prescribing resources including the BNF and BNF for Children.

Statement 2: *The General Practice Consultation*

A GP should be able to communicate clearly, sensitively and effectively, be committed to patient-centred medicine and have a clear understanding of what makes a good consultation and how it is achieved. This statement explains the importance of developing the effective communication and consultation skills that lie at the heart of general practice. As consulting is so central to being a GP, many of the skills involved are also covered by the core competences of general practice, such as person-centred care, described in Chapter 6, 'The core competences'.

The condensed skills

		☑ or score (1–5)
Consultation skills	Developing consultation skills typically associated with good doctor–patient communication, including sharing decisions with patients.	
IM&T skills	Keeping accurate, legible and contemporaneous patient records, and using the practice's records systems effectively.	
Negotiation skills	Negotiating effectively with patients or relatives and with colleagues over management and skills to limit consultation length when appropriate.	
Reflective skills	Undertaking self-appraisal through reflective logs and video recordings of consultations, and identifying learning needs from these; recognising, monitoring and managing emotions arising from the consultation.	
Team-working skills	Communicating with, delegating to, managing and supporting colleagues and staff.	
Telephone triage skills	Communicating and consulting effectively and safely via telephone and email.	

The condensed know-how

	☑ or score (1–5)
Common models of the consultation and how these models can be used to shape future consulting behaviour. **Tip:** *The common consultation models are summarised below.*	
Familiarity with the RCGP triaxial model: a biological, a psychological and a social component to every consultation. **Tip:** *More details of the triaxial model are available at www.gp-training.net.*	
How consulting behaviour and attitudes may vary with age, gender, ethnicity and the social background of the patient.	
Models of the process by which patients decide to consult, and how this can affect consulting outcomes. **Tip:** *Helman's 'Folk model of illness' (1981)[1] and Becker and Maiman's 'Health belief model' (1975)[2] are relevant to this.*	
How the doctor's agenda may conflict with the patient or relative's agenda (e.g. QoF targets, evidence-based medicine, public health responsibilities, child protection). **Tip:** *Always remember the central tenet of GP consulting: discover the patient's ideas, concerns and expectations.[3]*	
Roles and expertise of colleagues and other primary healthcare team members.	
Inter-professional boundaries of clinical responsibility and confidentiality. **Tip:** *Review the six Caldicott principles.[4]*	
A GP's professional roles and responsibilities towards the patient. **Tip:** *Read the GMC document* Good Medical Practice.[5]	
Resources to support patient education and information sharing, the role of expert patients. **Tip:** *For info on expert patients go to: www.expertpatients.nhs.uk.*	
Methods of making timely and appropriate referrals (e.g. using two-week wait).	

The condensed resources

The following table condenses six well-known consultation models:

Stott and Davis (1979)[6] – exceptional potential in each consultation	**Neighbour (1987)[7] – five-checkpoint model**
1. Managing the presenting complaint.	1. Connecting.
2. Managing ongoing problems.	2. Summarising.
3. Opportunistic health promotion.	3. Handover.
4. Modifying health-seeking behaviour.	4. Safety-netting.
	5. Housekeeping.

Pendleton *et al.* (1984, 2003)[3] – seven-tasks model	**Tuckett *et al.* (1985)[8] – meeting of two experts**
1. Define the reason for the patient's attendance (ideas, concerns and expectations).	● The consultation is a meeting between two experts.
2. Consider other problems.	● Doctors are experts in medicine.
3. Choose appropriate action.	● Patients are experts in their own illnesses.
4. Share understanding with the patient.	● Shared understanding is the aim.
5. Involve the patient in management decisions.	● Doctors should seek to understand the patient's beliefs.
6. Use time and resources well.	● Doctors should address explanations in terms of the patient's belief system.
7. Establish and maintain the doctor–patient relationship.	

Stewart *et al.* (1995, 2003)[9] – patient-centred clinical method	**Calgary–Cambridge observation guide (1996)[10] – stages of a consultation**
1. Exploring both the disease and the illness experience.	1. Initiating the session.
2. Understanding the whole person.	2. Gathering information.
3. Finding common ground.	3. Building the relationship.
4. Incorporating prevention and health promotion.	4. Explanation and planning.
5. Enhancing the patient–doctor relationship.	5. Closing the session.
6. Being realistic (with time and resources).	

- A useful summary of the common consultation models is available at www.trainer.org.uk.

- A large collection of printable information leaflets suitable for UK patients is available at www.patient.co.uk.

   The following methods are good for developing consultation skills:

- Learn a number of consultation models (Roger Neighbour's 'five-checkpoint model' from *The Inner Consultation*[7] is insightful for everyday consulting).

- Video your consultations – and force yourself to review them!

- Analyse consultations with a trainer or mentor. The new MRCGP consultation observation tool (COT) has been designed for this purpose (see Chapter 5, 'Succeeding at the new MRCGP'). Alternatively, try 'consultation mapping' (www.gp-training.net).

- The Calgary–Cambridge model[11] is a useful framework for exploring new consultation techniques.

- Role-play with actors or colleagues (remember: 'no pain, no gain!').

- Ask patients to give candid feedback at the end of the consultation.

- Sit in with an experienced GP and conduct joint surgeries with several GPs.

   Below is a list of some of the textbooks and publications that have been influential in the development of GP consulting skills, which are worth a read (a more extensive list is available in the full curriculum statement).

Berne E. *Games People Play* London: Penguin, 1964.

Goleman D. *Emotional Intelligence* London: Bloomsbury, 1996.

Neighbour R. *The Inner Consultation* Lancaster: MTP, 1987.

Pendleton D, Schofield T, Tate P, Havelock P, *The New Consultation: developing doctor–patient communication* Oxford: Radcliffe Medical Press, 2003.

Stott N C and Davis R H. The exceptional potential in each primary care consultation *Journal of the Royal College of General Practitioners* 1979; **29**: 201–5.

Tate P. *The Doctor's Communication Handbook* (fourth edn). Oxford: Radcliffe Medical Press, 2002.

Usherwood T. *Understanding the Consultation* Buckingham: Open University Press, 1999.

Statement 3.1: *Clinical Governance*

A GP must place the needs of patients before his or her personal convenience or interests. Every GP must understand the principles of clinical governance and use them in his or her everyday professional practice. The main aim of clinical governance is to improve the quality and accountability of health care, to identify and respond to poor practice, and to create a supportive culture with good teamwork, underpinned by clinical audit.

The condensed Skills

		☑ or score (1–5)
Audit skills	Aim to conduct at least one eight-stage clinical audit and one significant event audit during your training. **Tip:** *The eight-stage audit process is shown below.*	
Change management skills	Planning and implementing change in the practice (e.g. introducing a new guideline).	
Feedback skills	Giving and receiving feedback effectively. **Tip:** *Familiarise yourself with the Pendleton rules[3] for giving effective feedback (see Chapter 4, 'Teaching the curriculum').*	

The condensed know-how

	☑ or score (1–5)

Quality improvement systems:

- The general principles, methods and concepts of quality assurance
- NHS quality improvement systems, at national and local levels
- Issues around inequalities in health care and involvement of patients to assist in service planning
- Methods for ascertaining the views of patient.

Tip: *Conduct a PDSA cycle (plan–do–study–act).[12]*

☑ or score
(1–5)

Leadership:

- The rationale for a practice clinical governance lead, their key relationships and responsibilities.

Implementing evidence-based practice:

- Definition of clinical guidelines, their development, knowing how to assess the quality of a clinical guideline, kite-marking, differences between a guideline and a protocol.

Tip: *The NHS Clinical Governance Support Team website contains an 'About CG' section with a glossary that defines these terms: www.cgsupport.nhs.uk.*

Dissemination of good practice, ideas and innovation:

- The issues in involving patients from backgrounds that reflect the local population
- Models of change management
- Methods of obtaining feedback.

Tip: *Try to attend a meeting of the clinical governance committee of your local Primary Care Organisation (e.g. PCT [Primary Care Trust]).*

Clinical Risk Reduction and detection of adverse events:

- Common medical errors
- The causes of delayed referrals
- Recording significant events
- The issues around patient access to their records.

Tip: *Find out about the Access to Medical Reports and Data Protection Acts.*

Learning lessons from complaints:

- The NHS complaints systems and optimal methods for learning from errors and dealing with patient complaints
- The issues around engaging patients in the care of others, e.g. the Expert Patient Programme
- The issues around involving lay people in the improvement of health services and patient groups.

Tip: *Risk management is covered in condensed statement 3.2:* Patient Safety.

Addressing poor clinical performance:

- Methods of diagnosis and management, performance indicators, local procedures
- When it is appropriate to raise concerns and how to access local complaint and doctor support systems.

Continued over

☑ or score
(1–5)

Professional development:

- The relationship between clinical governance, continuing professional development, appraisal and revalidation.

High-quality data:

- Defining and assessing the performance of a GP and a practice
- Clinical audit cycle
- Critical appraisal skills (for evaluating performance indicators and determinants of variation in performance data.

Professional standards:

- The codes and standards that apply to GPs and primary care; professional, regulatory, national, NHS, legal and local standards for clinical and professional conduct.

Tip: *Read the General Medical Council's* Good Medical Practice[5] *or the RCGP's* Good Medical Practice for General Practitioners.[13]

The condensed resources

- The Clinical Governance Support Team provides information, guidance and assists organisations in successfully implementing clinical governance: www.cgsupport.nhs.uk.

- NHS Quality Improvement Scotland (NHS QIS) is the lead organisation for improving the quality of health care in Scotland: www.nhshealthquality.org.

The eight-stage clinical audit cycle

1. Describe the reason for choice of audit, considering the potential for change and relevance of the audit to the practice.

2. Identify the audit criteria, ensuring the criteria chosen are relevant to the audit subject and are justified by relevant evidence.

3. Set the audit standards; this involves setting appropriate targets and a suitable timescale.

4. Prepare and plan the audit, recording evidence of teamwork and discussion where appropriate.

5. Complete the first data collection, comparing the results against the standards.

6. Implement the changes to be evaluated, with examples described.

7. Complete the second data collection and compare the results with the first data collection and the standards.

8. Describe the conclusions, including any barriers to change and a summary of the issues learned.

Statement 3.2: *Patient Safety*

Addressing the safety of patients systematically across both the practice and wider NHS can have a positive impact on the quality and efficiency of patient care. Patient safety is a relatively young field and GPs will require ongoing training throughout their career. GPs are in a strong position to positively influence the safety culture within their practice and its development as a learning organisation. The knowledge and application of risk assessment tools must become part of a GP's core set of skills and, whenever change occurs in their working environment, GPs should assess the risks of this change and plan accordingly.

The condensed skills

		☑ or score (1–5)
Communication skills	Communicating openly, listening and taking patients' concerns seriously, and telling patients fully, honestly and compassionately about incidents when they occur.	
Reflective skills	Identifying the limitations of your own skills in risk management and when the skills risk assessment professionals should be called upon.	
Risk assessment skills	Carrying out a risk assessment and using a risk matrix.	
	Tip: *The Health and Safety Executive (HSE) website has a useful guide on carrying out a risk assessment: www.hse.gov.uk.*	
Team-working skills	Sharing and implementing lessons within the team from the analysis of patient safety incidents.	

The condensed know-how

	☑ or score (1–5)
How organisations and individuals can learn to be vigilant for patient safety incidents, how a change in clinical behaviour and/or practice systems influences patient safety and the impact of the GP's working environment on risk. **Tip:** *Participate in risk management meetings and discussions in the practice and consider how to develop a 'safety culture'.*	
Current clinical governance guidelines that impact on patient safety within a practice. **Tip:** *Consult the NPSA's 'Being Open policy' (www.npsa.nhs.uk) for advice on what to do when a patient safety incident occurs.*	
The basic principles of risk assessment and the elements of an appropriate infrastructure for risk management: • Creating a culture that is open and fair • Policies that commit the organisation to being open about serious incidents • Policies that state the actions that staff should take following an incident • Individual roles and accountability • The mechanism of investigating errors • Support for patients, family and staff • Staff training. **Tip:** *Identify the systems and processes set up in your practice to manage risk and compare these systems with those in the practices of your colleagues.*	
Tools that can be applied in risk management and patient safety issues. **Tip:** *Risk management tools are accessible from sites such as www.saferhealthcare.org.uk and the medical indemnity organisation websites.*	
How changes in the IT structure of the NHS will impact on the risk of patient safety incidents. **Tip:** *This relates to the different types of continuity of care, record keeping and the interface between primary and secondary care.*	
The criteria for when a root cause analysis or significant event audit should be performed (these criteria should include all incidents that have led to permanent harm or death). **Tip:** *Keep a log or diary of consecutive consultations one day per month and review any actual or potential safety incidents within those consultations.*	

Continued over

Reporting adverse incidents:

- How to assess an organisation's reporting and learning culture
- Systems for reporting patient safety incidents both locally and nationally.

Tip: *Familiarise yourself with the yellow-card system for reporting adverse drug events. Look in the back of the BNF or at www.yellowcard.gov.uk for more details.*

Significant event analysis (SEA):

- Consider the rationale for participation of the whole team in SEA and reasons for the inclusion or exclusion of different team members
- Identify methods of implementing solutions to reduce the risk of harm
- Discuss issues relevant to embedding any lessons learnt in the practice's working processes and systems
- Identify which other patient services may be affected by the same issues in future and how to share learning more widely.

Tip: *Write up a SEA from a patient seen during the general practice period of training. Reflect on the learning and consider whether reporting locally or nationally would be appropriate. Identify the measures that the practice takes to ensure that reports are dealt with fairly and that the appropriate learning and action take place.*

The role of the local Patient Advice and Liaison Service (PALS) or equivalent and how to contact them.

Tip: *Your local Primary Care Organisation (e.g. PCT) has a local PALS contact.*

Steps to facilitate safe multi-professional working with:

- Other practice team members
- Community pharmacists
- Community nurses and health visitors
- Community matrons and case managers
- Care programme approach
- Secondary care
- Social services.

Tip: *Consider a patient pathway in which a number of different healthcare professionals have been involved. Reflect on the safety issues arising from each interface between each provider and the ways in which these can be reduced (e.g. quality of communication, referral letters, handovers).*

How patient groups may be put at increased risk by virtue of their particular characteristics, such as language, literacy, culture and health beliefs.	
How the lessons of patient safety can be applied prospectively to doctor–patient interactions, especially through the identification and discussion of risk.	

The condensed resources

- The National Patient Safety Agency (NPSA) is responsible for improving quality of care through reporting, analysing and learning from patient safety incidents and 'near misses' involving NHS patients: www.npsa.nhs.uk.

- Significant event analysis (or audit) training tools are available from medical defence associations, NPSA and www.saferhealthcare.org.uk.

- The Medicines and Healthcare products Regulatory Agency is the government agency responsible for ensuring that medicines and medical devices are safe. Its website contains lots of information on patient safety as well as safety warnings, alerts, and how to report safety concerns: www.mhra.gov.uk.

- The Health and Safety Executive provides useful information on health and safety issues, and performing risk assessment: www.hse.gov.uk.

Statement 3.3: *Clinical Ethics and Values-Based Practice*

General practitioners, in common with all health professionals, must act in accordance with the ethical principles set out in professional codes of conduct. Ethical decision-making and behaviour require the application and interpretation of these principles within the specific context of general practice, taking into account the perspectives and values of all involved. General practitioners need to be able to justify their decisions with reference to both the clinical evidence and the moral and other values that inform those decisions. This is applicable across the whole curriculum and should be incorporated into all aspects of clinical practice, management and research.

The condensed skills

		☑ or score (1–5)
Moral reasoning skills	Considering the ethical dimension of every healthcare encounter.	
	Choosing an appropriate course of action and resolving opposing values, such as balancing conflicting duties to two individual patients who are members of the same family.	
Reflective skills	Recognising personal values and how these influence decision making and the ability to clarify and justify personal ethics.	

The condensed know-how

	☑ or score (1–5)
The professional ethical guidelines and legal frameworks within which healthcare decisions should be made. **Tip:** *Familiarise yourself with the GMC's document* Good Medical Practice.[5]	
Guidance on consent and confidentiality in the particular context of primary care and how co-morbidity or disease progression may affect decision-making capacity. **Tip:** *Find out about the recent changes introduced by the Mental Capacity Act 2005 and the new Lasting Power of Attorney.*	

	☑ or score (1–5)
Research evidence on the patient values that are likely to influence a given healthcare situation. **Tip:** *Consider Helman's 'Folk model of illness' (1981).*[1]	
The ethical issues raised by public health programmes and appropriate approaches to implementing these programmes.	
Frameworks of moral reasoning for facilitating the consideration of ethical issues and resolving conflicts of values. **Tip:** *Consider the 'big four' ethical principles (see below).*	
How to recognise and respond to a patient entering a terminal stage of illness, and the values that are important in managing this. **Tip:** *You can find out about living wills at www.livingwill.org.uk.*	
Potential ethical difficulties that might arise in practice and proactive strategies to prevent or reduce the likelihood of ethical conflicts arising for yourself and for patients. **Tip:** *Read your practice's policies on accepting gifts from patients and for ensuring financial probity within the practice.*	
Concepts of distributive justice that are used in resource allocation debates, the range of values that influence choices about healthcare provision.	
Understanding the obligation to use public resources in a prudent manner to benefit the whole community, plus morally relevant reasons for making decisions that balance individual patient needs with the needs of the wider community.	
How the values and beliefs prevalent in the local culture impact on patient care.	
How the social context of primary care frames the identification and resolution of ethical issues by GPs.	
The process for gaining ethics approval for research conducted in primary care. **Tip:** *Find out about the role of local Ethics Committees. The Central Office for Research Ethics Committees has more information: www.corec.org.uk.*	

The condensed resources

The 'big four' ethical principles form a useful basic theoretical framework for considering ethical issues:

Beneficence	**Non-maleficence**
Doing good	Doing no harm

Autonomy	**Justice**
Acting in accordance with an individual's right to be free, independent and self-directing	Acting in accordance with the principles of truth, reason, fairness and the law

The Medical Protection Society (www.medicalprotection.org) and the Medical Defence Union (www.the-mdu.com) offer information and advice on the key legal aspects relevant to general practice.

The General Medical Committee (GMC) has a statutory role to provide guidance to doctors on medical ethics and good practice. A core publication is *Good Medical Practice* (2006), which sets out the principles and values on which good practice is founded. It can be downloaded at: www.gmc-uk.org.

Statement 3.4: *Promoting Equality and Valuing Diversity*

Equality is creating a fairer society in which every person has the opportunity to fulfil his or her potential. Diversity is about recognising and valuing difference in its broadest sense. The principles of equality and diversity run through the whole curriculum and together are a central principle of modern patient care. The two are paired, as there can be no true equality of opportunity unless the value of diversity is also recognised.

Much of the learning associated with this curriculum statement concerns the development of attitudes and behaviours that promote equality and diversity. GPs have a professional duty to act in ways that recognise that people are in many ways different and not to discriminate against people because of these differences, and to acknowledge people's right to take responsibility for their health and to make their own health decisions.

The condensed skills

		☑ or score (1–5)
Assertiveness skills	Effectively challenging behaviour that infringes the rights of others and addressing discrimination, oppression and harassment against oneself and others.	
Communication skills	Communicating with patients from diverse backgrounds, providing information in ways that help people to exercise their individual rights.	
	Making effective use of the various interpreting and communications support services.	

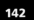

The condensed know-how

	☑ or score (1–5)

Procedures, policies and legislation appertaining to equality and diversity, including national law and international conventions relating to:

- Human rights (including children)
- Equality
- Anti-discriminatory practices
- Mental health
- Complaints and issue resolution
- Employment
- Disability.

Tip: *Talk to your practice manager about the steps your practice has taken to comply with the Disability Discrimination Act (with respect to both patients and staff).*

Employment and recruitment practices and workplace anti-discrimination legislation.

Tip: *Review your practice's employment policies and/or staff handbook.*

How differences in ethnicity and culture and individual and social context impact on health, illness and health care.

Tip: *Find out how to access your local translation services e.g. www.languageline.co.uk.*

Issues around migration, demography of cultural groups, experience of socio-economic disadvantage and patterns of illness and disease.

Poverty as a cause of poor health and poor health as a cause of poverty.

Tip: *Look up the main findings of the Acheson Inquiry into health inequalities (1998)*[14] *which is available at: www.archive.official-documents.co.uk.*

Appropriate knowledge of ethnic and cultural behaviour including specific practical knowledge (e.g. nutrition, naming systems, religion, attitudes toward illness, death, and pregnancy).

Tip: *If you work in a community with a low level of cultural diversity, this does not mean you won't need to devote as much effort to learning about various cultural groups – in fact you will have to try harder to acquire this knowledge as your experience of meeting such patients will be more limited than GPs in more diverse communities.*

Awareness of specific issues around the care of homeless people.

Awareness of specific issues around the care of asylum seekers and refugees.

The condensed resources

The Commission for Racial Equality issues a code of practice for general practice: www.cre.gov.uk.

There is a strong base of legislation within the UK central to the promotion of equality and valuing of diversity. Here are some of the more important acts relevant to general practice:

- Equal Pay Act 1970
- Sex Discrimination Act 1975 and 1986
- Mental Health Act 1983
- Gender Reassignment Regulations 1999
- Race Relations Act 1976 and Race Relations (Amendment) Act 2000
- Disability Discrimination Act 1995
- Employment Rights Act 1996
- Human Rights Act 1998
- Employment Relations Act 1999
- Maternity and Paternity Leave Regulations 1999
- Part-Time Workers Regulations 2000
- Employment Act 2002
- European Union Employment Directive and European Union Race and Ethnic Origin Directive
- Mental Capacity Act 2005.

Statement 3.5: *Evidence-Based Practice*

Evidence-based health care means using a rigorous and scientific approach to appraise evidence (from a range of sources) to benefit individual patients and to improve the delivery of health care. GPs must be able to interpret scientific information in order to provide patients with information appropriate to them and their circumstances. A GP must learn the skills required to search for the 'best evidence', to appraise it critically and to apply it appropriately to all areas of general practice.

The condensed knowledge

		☑ or score (1–5)
Basic statistics	Absolute risk (AR) and absolute risk reduction (ARR).	
	Hazard ratio (HR).	
	Incidence and prevalence.	
	Number needed to harm (NNH) and number needed to treat (NNT).	
	Odds and odds ratio (OR).	
	Pre- and post-test probability.	
	Positive predictive value (PPV) and negative predictive value (NPV).	
	Relative risk (RR) and relative risk reduction (RRR).	
	Specificity and sensitivity.	
Critical appraisal	Appropriateness of prospective and retrospective studies.	
	Bias, inclusion and exclusion criteria, and representativeness of samples.	
	Common tests used to analyse parametric data (e.g. awareness of t-tests, analysis of variance, multiple regression) and non-parametric data (e.g. awareness of chi-squared, Mann–Whitney U tests).	
	Confidence intervals, probability and correlation coefficients.	

		☑ or score (1–5)
Critical appraisal	Methods used to validate qualitative research (e.g. triangulation, saturation).	
	Reliability, validity and generalisability of findings.	
	Research methodologies and their appropriate use (see condensed statement 3.6: *Research and Academic Activity*).	

The condensed skills

		☑ or score (1–5)
Communication skills	Communicating risks and benefits in a way that is meaningful to patients.	
Consulting skills	Enhancing patient concordance with evidence-based lifestyle and therapeutic interventions.	
	Using the doctor–patient relationship to reconcile the patient's personal objectives with the available solutions to his or her medical problems.	
Critical appraisal skills	Searching, evaluating, interpreting and applying best evidence and offering patients healthcare choices based on this evidence, tailored according to the patient's personal values and motivation.	

The condensed know-how

	☑ or score (1–5)
Reliable sources of the best possible evidence to base decisions and to inform patients of the 'best possible' way to navigate the healthcare system.	
Basic statistics and how to evaluate a scientific paper. **Tip:** *There are lots of books on basic statistics. Or look at www.cebm.net.*	
Factors affecting the efficacy of evidence-based interventions: ● Concordance with therapeutic aims ● Continuity of care and a long-term relationship ● The role of the doctor–patient relationship. **Tip:** *A combination of evidence-based treatments is not necessarily an evidence-based approach in itself. Interactions between the various interventions may affect efficacy.*	
Awareness of the scarcity of evidence derived from a patient's perspective and that most studies don't include quality-of-life measures. **Tip:** *Consider the relative merits of quantitative and qualitative research.*	
The limitations of evidence in patients with chronic disease in primary care, especially as much evidence excludes patients with significant co-morbidity.	
The issue of health inequalities when applying evidence to minorities and awareness that the majority of evidence-based guidelines do not include ethnicity or socio-economic status as risk factors. **Tip:** *Always check to see if the population in a study is applicable to your own practice's population.*	
The limitations of separating scientific and non-scientific approaches to health and the issues arising when patients differ from their doctors in the value they attach to medical evidence. **Tip:** *A patient's objectives in a consultation are often driven by his or her values, although the solutions a GP can offer are often 'value-neutral', or based on the medical profession's values. For example, an evidence-based guideline for diagnosing headache is unlikely to offer much comfort to an anxious patient whose relative recently died of a stroke.*	

The condensed resources

- The National Library for Health (www.library.nhs.uk) contains an excellent collection of resources on EBM. Among the most useful resources are:

  - The Cochrane Library: www.thecochranelibrary.com

  - Bandolier: www.jr2.ox.ac.uk/bandolier

  - The National Library for Health's 'question-answering service' is available free to GPs. Its team seeks to answer EBM questions that health professionals have been unable to answer for themselves: www.clinicalanswers.nhs.uk

- The Oxford Centre for Evidence-Based Medicine: www.cebm.net

- The NICE guidelines: www.nice.org.uk

- The SIGN guidelines: www.sign.ac.uk

- Trisha Greenhalgh's book *How to Read a Paper: the basics of evidence based medicine* (Blackwell Publishing, 2006) provides a good introduction to evidence-based medicine.

Statement 3.6: *Research and Academic Activity*

General practice is an academic discipline at the heart of decision making in the NHS. Academic activity involves all GPs to some extent and comprises not only research, but also teaching and reflective practice. Research *in* primary care provides the GP with the means to test and improve clinical practice, evaluate innovative models of service delivery and to understand population data. Research *on* primary care provides the means to improve organisation of services and to question local beliefs or behaviours on the basis of population data.

The condensed knowledge

		☑ or score (1–5)
Research methodologies	Case-control studies.	
	Cohort studies.	
	Interviews, focus groups and questionnaires.	
	Meta-analysis.	
	Narrative-based research.	
	Pilot studies.	
	Qualitative research.	
	Quantitative research.	
	Randomised controlled trials.	
	Systematic reviews.	

The condensed skills

		☑ or score (1–5)
Research skills	Accessing evidence.	
Tip: *Look at the Centre for Evidence-Based Medicine's website for tips on how to develop these skills: www.cebm.net*	Basic statistics.	
	Critical appraisal.	
	Evaluating ethical issues and the need to have projects approved through research governance committees.	
	Implementing change in clinical practice.	
	Prioritising relevant information.	
	Problem framing.	

The condensed know-how

	☑ or score (1–5)

The research process:

1. Develop a research question

2. Identify appropriate methods from a range of designs

3. Be able to draw up a questionnaire

4. Demonstrate basic quantitative and qualitative data-analysis skills

5. Draw appropriate conclusions

6. Summarise results.

Tip: *The RCGP website contains information for GPs interested in carrying out research: www.rcgp.org.uk/research.*

How to provide patients involved in research with full information and informed consent.

Tip: *The Central Office for Research Ethics Committees has more information on this and the other ethical aspects of research: www.corec.org.uk.*

Patients' right to choose whether or not to accept new interventions.

Tip: *Consider the principles of informed consent and patient autonomy (see condensed statement 3.3:* Clinical Ethics and Values-Based Practice*).*

Confidentiality and Data Protection Act requirements.

Tip: *The Information Commissioner provides advice and tools on the Data Protection Act: www.ico.gov.uk.*

Quantitative methods of research (such as randomised controlled trials).

Qualitative methods of research (such as 'grounded theory').

The range of resources available from postgraduate and university departments.

Tip: *Your local continuing professional development (CPD) tutor should be able to provide information on local academic resources.*

The condensed resources

- The EBM journal Bandolier contains a glossary explaining key research terms: www.jr2.ox.ac.uk/bandolier/glossary.html.

- RDLearning contains a database of health-related training courses available in the UK with a particular emphasis on research. The database covers workshops, conferences and short courses from higher-education institutions, professional bodies, research networks and training organisations: www.rdlearning. org.uk.

- Trisha Greenhalgh's book *How to Read a Paper: the basics of evidence-based medicine* (Blackwell Publishing, 2006) covers basic medical statistics.

Statement 3.7: *Teaching, Mentoring and Clinical Supervision*

Successful teaching involves developing a range of methods for facilitating a learner's learning process. Teaching, mentoring and supervision are core activities of general practice and, at some stage, every GP will have some form of teaching, mentoring or supervisory role. GPs need to develop learner-centred strategies to encourage learner autonomy and provide support as mentors. The skills involved in consulting with patients are similar to the skills required for effective teaching. GP trainees are likely to be increasingly involved in teaching in the future, whether this takes the form of leading seminars for other trainees or supervising Foundation Programme doctors.

The condensed skills

		☑ or score (1–5)
Adult learning skills	Carrying out an educational needs analysis and designing an educational programme appropriate to the learner.	
	Tip: *Chapter 4, 'Teaching the curriculum', contains information on how to do this.*	
Feedback skills	Asking for and learning from feedback on performance as a teacher and how to give effective feedback to a colleague.	
	Tip: *The annual appraisal has a section on teaching to ask for documented feedback and record this in your portfolio.*	
IM&T skills	Making use of information management and technology in teaching.	
	Tip: *Every training practice should have access to a projector for PowerPoint presentations.*	
Mentoring skills	The ability to ask for, organise, receive and also give forms of mentorship and supervision appropriate to each career stage.	

Continued over

		☑ or score (1–5)
Presentation skills	Delivering a presentation clearly and effectively, identifying the needs of the audience, tailoring the presentation to those needs and encouraging active involvement.	
	Tip: *Give a short presentation to your training group; ask them to give you feedback and record it in your learning portfolio.*	
Teaching skills	Planning and structuring a teaching episode (activity) appropriately for the learners concerned and facilitating the learning of a small group.	
	Tip: *Training programmes should include a self-directed element to help trainees develop these skills.*	

The condensed know-how

	☑ or score (1–5)
Principles of adult learning theory.	
Tip: *These are described in Chapter 3, 'Learning the curriculum'.*	
Individual learning styles and preferences.	
Tip: *Complete a learning style questionnaire to identify your learning preferences (e.g. Honey and Mumford,[15] which divides learners into theorists, activists, pragmatists and reflectors – see Chapter 4, 'Teaching the curriculum').*	
The principles of a learner-centred approach to teaching.	
The steps in an educational needs analysis.	
Tip: *For ways of identifying learning needs, see Chapter 3, 'Learning the curriculum'.*	
The definitions of inter-professional and multi-professional learning.	
The nature and purpose of mentoring and clinical supervision, and the different forms of these (both formal and informal).	

	☑ or score (1–5)
The relationship between teaching and reflective practice. **Tip:** *Keep a reflective diary to record significant consultations.*	
Ways of establishing a culture of teaching and learning within a practice. **Tip:** *www.gp-training.net has more information on learning organisations.*	
Models of teaching (didactic, Socratic, etc.). **Tip:** *See Chapter 4, 'Teaching the curriculum', for some common teaching models.*	

The condensed resources

- The Honey and Mumford learning styles questionnaire is available from: www.peterhoney.com.

- The Myers–Briggs Personality Indicator is available from: www.myersbriggs.org.

- Chapters 3 and 4, 'Learning the curriculum' and 'Teaching the curriculum', contain lots of information and advice that are relevant to this statement.

Statement 4.1: *Management in Primary Care*

GPs work in primary-care teams, in practices that are becoming increasingly large and complex organisations, offering a growing range of services to patients. GPs must be equipped with the knowledge and skills to enable them to take on managerial responsibility and to actively involve health professionals and patients in the delivery of health care. Management is an activity that involves planning, allocation of resources, coordinating the work of others, employing and motivating staff, monitoring output and taking responsibility. GPs who manage inevitably require leadership skills and in a high-performing organisation every member will take responsibility for ensuring its success.

The condensed skills

		☑ or score (1–5)
Appraisal skills	Interviewing and staff appraisal skills (to be able to conduct an appraisal interview with staff and/or colleagues).	
Delegation skills	Delegating tasks effectively and safely. **Tip:** *Delegated tasks should be SMART: Specific, Measurable, Agreed, Realistic and Time-bound.*	
Leadership skills	Leading a team effectively. **Tip:** *Some leadership models are described at www.gp-training.net.*	
Management skills	Organising and running an effective meeting, using time management and project management skills (to plan and manage a project in the practice according to a timescale). **Tip:** *Identify a project that you can plan and manage in your practice (e.g. setting up a new chronic disease clinic).*	
Negotiation skills	Negotiating effectively with colleagues, staff and patients. **Tip:** BMJ Careers Focus *has a useful article on negotiation skills:*[16] *Crockett P and Hull A. How to negotiate effectively* BMJ Career Focus *2003;* ***326****: s49a, http://careerfocus.bmj.com.*	

	☑ or score (1–5)
Team-working skills Working as an effective member of a team and coordinating a team-based approach. **Tip:** *The Multi-Source Feedback tool of the new MRCGP Workplace-Based Assessment tests this skill.*	

The condensed know-how

	☑ or score (1–5)
The roles of the various members of the primary-care team. **Tip:** *Make a list of all the people who work in your primary-care team and their respective roles.*	
Factors that motivate staff and the role of team dynamics in the functioning of an organisation. **Tip:** *Maslow's Hierarchy of Needs[17] and McClelland's motivational needs theory[18] are useful models for understanding what motivates different people.*	
Ways of contributing to staff development and training.	
Strategies for effective communication within the practice organisation. **Tip:** *Consider which type of meetings and other communication strategies are used in your practice. How reliable and effective are they?*	
Methods of evaluating your own preference for roles within teams and in interactions with others. **Tip:** *Learn about the Belbin team roles.[19] Which role(s) do you adopt?*	
Possible management structures of a practice, including how decisions are made and how responsibilities are distributed. **Tip:** *Try mapping out your practice's management structure. Compare it with other local practices. If you can't easily map it out, what does that imply?*	
The duties, rights and responsibilities of a GP as an employer and the fundamentals of employment law. **Tip:** *This is a good topic for a tutorial with the practice manager.*	
The health and occupational safety responsibilities of a GP (either as an employer or co-worker). **Tip:** *See the condensed statement 3.2:* Patient Safety.	

Continued over

☑ **or score**
(1–5)

The recruitment process and selection of staff or colleagues in accordance with the law relating to equal opportunities.

Tip: *Ask if you can be involved in the recruitment and selection of a new staff member (e.g. a new receptionist).*

The principles of medical device management and the use of the Adverse Incident Centre for reporting device-related adverse incidents.

The process of change and the factors that influence it (in teams and organisations).

Tip: *Find out how to perform a SWOT analysis (Strengths, Weaknesses, Opportunities, Threats).*

Processes and mechanisms of quality improvement in the practice.

Principles of leadership (in the NHS), and ways your own attitudes and feelings can determine how you manage and lead.

Tip: *BMJ Career Focus contains articles on management and leadership: http://careerfocus.bmj.com.*

Practice-based commissioning – the process of how services are commissioned and the conflicts of interest that might arise in the commissioning and provision of services, and how to include patients in the design of services.

Tip: *The Public Health Resource Unit (www.phru.nhs.uk) provides educational resources to help GPs to develop practice-based commissioning skills.*

Ways to establish the expectations that patients, carers and families have of their practice and local primary-care services.

Tip: *Find out if your practice has a patient forum or newsletter and consider other ways of obtaining patient feedback.*

Ways of involving patients in the management of the practice and delivery of local primary-care services and the positive benefits of involving patients in the systems of healthcare provision and quality improvement.

The various means by which general practitioners are contracted (e.g. General Medical Services [GMS], Personal Medical Services [PMS], etc.) and the key features of the contractual agreements (e.g. global sum, QoF, enhanced services) and how the organisation of a practice varies with its setting (e.g. rural, inner city, urban, academic, dispensing).

Tip: *Information on the various GP contracts (GMS, PMS, etc.) and other relevant practice management issues (e.g. practice-based commissioning) can be found on the Department of Health website (www.dh.gov.uk) and the British Medical Association website (www.bma.org.uk).*

☑ **or score**
(1–5)

The financial aspects of a practice, such as sources of income and expenditure, management of funding, use of premises, marketing, and the interpretation of accounts and factors affecting profitability.

Tip: *Information of practice finances is available at www.healthcarerepublic.com/practice.*

Alternative ways in which health care may be delivered in the community (e.g. nurse-led clinics, case management) and how variation in resources and facilities may affect the delivery of health care.

The important national and local strategies for health care (e.g. National Service Frameworks, NHS Plans, etc.) and the current UK priorities and guidelines that influence service design and delivery.

Tip: *National Service Frameworks are available at www.library.nhs.uk.*

Ethical aspects relating to management and leadership in primary health care, e.g. approaches to use of resources, rationing, and involving the public and patients in decision making.

The condensed resources

- The NHS Modernisation Agency legacy website offers tools and advice on managing change in the NHS: www.wise.nhs.uk.

- First Practice Management provides a range of resources to support medical practice managers: www.firstpracticemanagement.co.uk.

- A collection of generic educational resources on teamwork, leadership and business skills is available at www.businessballs.com.

Statement 4.2: *Information Management and Technology*

GPs increasingly rely on electronic patient records and electronic communication to keep accurate and searchable clinical records, and to fulfil contractual requirements. This requires an under-standing of the principles of good electronic record keeping and a good knowledge of clinical coding systems. Current NHS initiatives will have a major effect as paper records are phased out and GPs must be aware of the risks of inaccurate, incomplete or ambiguous health data. All GP trainees will be expected to develop IT skills to at least European Computer Driving Licence standard.

The condensed skills

		☑ or score (1–5)
Clinical IM&T skills	Using the practice clinical system for tasks such as prescribing, entering clinical data, processing pathology results and referrals. This includes: • Using templates for the management of chronic disease and assessing risk • Using recall systems within the practice to the benefit of patient care • Using inter-agency systems such as pathology links and GP-to-GP record transfer • Using the computer in the consultation whilst maintaining rapport with the patient • Using NHS electronic booking systems to tailor healthcare provision to the needs of the individual patient. **Tip:** *Arrange a tutorial on your practice system and how to use Choose and Book.*	

	☑ or score (1–5)

| **Generic IM&T skills** | The RCGP recommends that GPs should have reached the standard of the European Computer Driving Licence (ECDL) by the end of their training. The seven modules that make up the ECDL are: <ul><li>Basic concepts of IT</li><li>Using the computer and managing files</li><li>Word processing</li><li>Spreadsheets</li><li>Databases</li><li>Presentations</li><li>Information and Communication.</li></ul> **Tip:** *For more information see www.ecdl.nhs.uk.* | |
| **IT search skills** | Finding the best evidence in practice. This includes: <ul><li>Using expert and web-based information systems, e.g. MENTOR and PRODIGY</li><li>Searching the internet for medical and scientific information including MEDLINE and the National Electronic Library for Health (www.library.nhs.uk).</li><li>Using IM&T to develop and maintain continuing learning and quality improvement.</li></ul> **Tip:** *Arrange a training session at your local NHS healthcare library on literature search techniques.* | |

The condensed know-how

	☑ or score (1–5)

| How clinical coding systems are used and their role in effective record keeping. **Tip:** *Find out about Read codes and SNOMED codes.* | |
| The connection between good data entry and improved patient health outcomes. **Tip:** *Consider the role of IM&T in maintaining continuity of care.* | |

Continued over

☑ **or score**
(1–5)

Ways information recorded in the practice clinical system may be shared with different health professionals and organisations to coordinate patient care, and the information governance and privacy obligations relating to the sharing of electronic records, and the central storage of health information.

Tip: *Read your practice's Freedom of Information, Data Protection and confidentiality policies.*

How to use reports from clinical systems for personal/practice audit and data analysis, and to improve the quality and usefulness of the medical record.

How to facilitate patient access to his or her medical record, the relevant rules and to enhance patient understanding of privacy and the consent issues concerning the shared electronic health record.

Tip: *Find out about the responsibilities of a GP under the Medical Reports Act.*

How to use IM&T to gain an understanding of the health needs of communities through the epidemiological characteristics of their population.

The main NHS IM&T initiatives and strategies, and the implications of these for the local health service.

Tip: *Familiarise yourself with the issues around recent initiatives such as Choose and Book, Electronic Prescribing, GP-to-GP records transfer and the Electronic Care Record (ECR).*

The importance of practice- and community-based information in the quality assurance of each doctor's practice.

Ways of using IM&T to access community-based resources, e.g. voluntary organisations and self-help groups.

Tip: *www.patient.co.uk has patient information leaflets and links to self-help groups and patient organisations.*

Ways of ensuring that the use of IM&T does not conflict with their holistic and patient-centred approach to patient care.

Tip: *Consider how a QoF alert system may affect a consultation.*

Awareness of the different computer systems used in practices.

Tip: *Arrange to visit a practice that use a different computer system and ask someone there to give you a brief run through the system.*

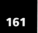

☑ or score
(1–5)

How context affects the ways in which record entries are understood and interpreted.	
Ethical and legal aspects of clinical practice relating to IM&T, e.g. security, confidentiality, use of information for insurance company use.	
Tip: *You should understand a GP's responsibilities under the Data Protection Act, Freedom of Information Act and Computer Misuse Act, and the consent and ethical issues raised by the Electronic Patient Record.*	

The condensed resources

- Information on the European Computer Driving Licence and essential IT skills for NHS staff can be obtained from www.ecdl.nhs.uk.

- The Information Commissioner is responsible for policing the Data Protection Act: www.ico.gov.uk.

- The Freedom of Information Act website contains useful information and resources for GPs: www.foi.nhs.uk.

- Connecting for Health is the organisation responsible for delivering the National Programme for IT and offers information on the Electronic Care Record: www.connectingforhealth.nhs.uk.

- Other relevant legislation is the Access to Medical Reports Act 1998 and the Computer Misuse Act 1990, both available on the Office of Public Sector Information website at www.opsi.gov.uk.

Statement 5: *Healthy People: promoting health and preventing disease*

GPs provide the link between individual health care and care for the local community. GPs must develop the skills to help people to self-care, via a range of approaches. This should be done as a partnership, recognising that the patient should make the necessary choices, decisions and take the actions themselves. During the consultation, there are opportunities to discuss healthy living with the patient and for the early detection of illness.

A competent GP must provide appropriate diagnostic, therapeutic and preventive services to individuals and to his or her registered population. A GP must, therefore, understand the concepts of health, function and quality of life as well as models of disease. These include health promotion and preventive activities, risk management and issues of cost-efficiency and rationing. Gaining a good understanding of health inequalities, and the strategies to address these, is an important aspect of GP training.

The condensed skills

		☑ or score (1–5)
Communication skills	Communicating risk effectively to the patient and their family.	
Consultation skills	Promoting health on an individual basis as part of the consultation and judging when a patient will be receptive to the concept of self-care.	
Negotiation skills	Reaching a shared understanding with the patient of common problems and their management (including self management strategies), so that the patient is enabled to look after their own health.	

The condensed know-how

	☑ or score (1–5)
The concepts of health and disease. **Tip:** *Review the WHO definitions at www.who.int.*	
The principles of prevention and preventive strategies, and the scientific backgrounds of public health, epidemiology and preventive healthcare. **Tip:** *Visit the Bandolier website: www.jr2.ox.ac.uk/bandolier/glossary.html.*	
The concepts of incidence and prevalence. **Tip:** *These are defined in Chapter 6, 'The core competences' (3.1a).*	
How to assess an individual patient's risk factors and the risk factors for disease, including alcohol and substance abuse, accidents, child abuse, diet, exercise, genetics, occupation, social deprivation and sexual behaviour.	
The role of health promotion and disease prevention programmes. **Tip:** *Information on screening programmes can be found on the NHS screening website: www.screening.nhs.uk.*	
The principles of immunisation and vaccination, the UK's immunisation programmes and the benefits and risks of immunisation. **Tip:** *The Green Book is the UK immunisation reference text (available at www.dh.gov.uk).*	
The benefits and risks of screening programmes, UK screening programmes, how to interpret evidence about a screening programme and decide whether it is worthwhile – for individuals or for groups. **Tip:** *Review the Wilson and Junger criteria[20] for screening programmes (see below).*	
The role of the public health specialist and how and when to access specialist public health advice. **Tip:** *The Faculty for Public Health of the Royal College of Physicians sets the standards for specialists in public health: www.fphm.org.uk.*	
The roles of the other professionals involved in public health, e.g. school nurses, health visitors and public health specialists. **Tip:** *Consider spending a day attached to some of these professionals.*	
The role of the GP and the primary healthcare team in health promotion activities in the community. **Tip:** *NICE have issued a Public Health Intervention guideline on physical activity that covers some of these issues (www.nice.org.uk).*	

Continued over

	☑ or score (1–5)
How to use routinely available data to describe the health of the local population, compare it with that of other populations, and identify localities or groups with poor health within it.	
How to undertake a needs assessment of a target group of patients.	
The principles of health surveillance and how it helps with planning of health services, providing alerts for contingency planning and for monitoring the equitable distribution of health care. **Tip:** *Current UK Child Health Surveillance policy can be found in* Health for All Children (*2003*).[21]	
The concept of risk and communicating risk. **Tip:** *There is an excellent BMJ theme issue on this topic:* BMJ Vol. 327, No. 7417 (*www.bmj.com*).	
The effects of smoking, alcohol and drugs on the patient and their family. **Tip:** *There is a NICE guideline on Smoking Cessation* (*www.nice.org.uk*).	
The causes of potential tension between the GP's health promotion role and the patient's own agenda.	
Behavioural change models (approaches to behavioural change and their relevance to health promotion and self-care). **Tip:** *Review Prochaska and DiClemente's 'cycle of change' model.*[22]	
The interrelationships between health and social care including the wider determinants of health within communities, e.g. housing, employment and education.	
The impact of poverty, genetics, ethnicity, geography, culture, the workplace and local epidemiology on an individual and a local community's health. **Tip:** *See condensed statement 3.4:* Promoting Equality and Valuing Diversity.	
The impact of inequalities and discrimination on health and the 'inverse care law' and the importance of involving the public and communities in improving health and reducing inequalities. **Tip:** *Tudor Hart, a GP, first described the Inverse Care Law in 1971.*[23]	

The condensed resources

- The UK immunisation schedules can be found in the Green Book: www.dh.gov.uk/en/Policyandguidance/Healthandsocial-caretopics/Greenbook/DH_4097254.

- Lots of information about screening can be found on the UK National Screening Committee website: www.nsc.nhs.uk.

- The King's Fund is a charitable foundation that publishes reports and policy documents, many of which are relevant to issues around health inequalities: www.kingsfund.org.uk.

The 10 Wilson and Junger criteria for a screening programme[20]

1. Is the disease an important public health problem?
2. Is there an effective treatment for localised disease?
3. Are facilities for further diagnosis and treatment available?
4. Is there an identifiable latent or early symptomatic stage of disease?
5. Is the technique to be used for screening effective?
6. Are the tests acceptable to the population?
7. Is the natural history of the disease known?
8. Is there a strategy for determining which patients should and should not be treated?
9. Is the cost of screening acceptable?
10. Is effective treatment available and does management of cases in the early stages have a favourable impact on prognosis?

Statement 6: *Genetics in Primary Care*

Genetics is a rapidly evolving area of medicine that, in particular, requires GPs to keep their skills and knowledge up to date. About one in 10 patients seen in primary care have a disorder with a genetic component. GPs must provide support and advice to patients and families with, or at risk of, genetic conditions.

Consideration of the family history is particularly important for identifying those at risk of cancer, cardiovascular disease and diabetes, as is an understanding of the genetic aspects of antenatal and newborn screening. GPs play a key role in identifying patients and families who would benefit from referral to specialist genetic services and, as genetic conditions are often multi-systemic, coordinating patient care with other health services.

The condensed knowledge

		☑ or score (1–5)
Symptoms	Symptoms and signs of genetic conditions vary widely, particularly in autosomal dominant conditions where symptoms may vary in number and severity between affected patients within the same family (e.g. variability of expression in neurofibromatosis). Anxiety about a family history of a disease, for example breast cancer, is also a common presentation.	
Conditions	*Tip: Clinical information on the conditions listed below is available at GPNotebook (www.gpnotebook.co.uk).* Examples of common chromosome anomalies: • Down's syndrome • Turner's syndrome • Klinefelter's syndrome • Translocations.	

		☑ or score (1–5)
Conditions	Autosomal dominant single-gene disorders: • Adult polycystic kidney disease • Neurofibromatosis • Huntington's disease • Hypercholesterolaemia.	
	Recessive single-gene disorders: • Cystic fibrosis • Haemoglobinopathies (sickle-cell disease, thalassaemias) • Haemochromatosis.	
	X-linked single-gene disorders: • Duchenne and Becker muscular dystrophies • Haemophilia A • Fragile X.	
	Disorders with a genetic component (e.g. bipolar disorder, cerebrovascular disease, cardiovascular disease, Alzheimer's, asthma).	
	Common familial cancers (e.g. breast, colon).	
	Conditions exhibiting variable inheritance patterns (e.g. inherited forms of deafness, muscular dystrophies).	
Investigation	How to draw and interpret a family tree and recognise basic patterns of inheritance, and knowledge of basic genetic tests.	
	Tip: *You can find out how to draw a 'pedigree' tree at www.clingensoc.org/Docs/Standards/CGSPedigree.pdf.*	
Treatment	Varies depending on the individual disease but includes, for example, regular surveillance or family-planning options.	
Basic knowledge	DNA as genetic material and how mutations and variants contribute to human disease.	
	Patterns of inheritance: single gene, chromosomal and multifactorial.	
	How to access genetic information, for example from regional genetics centres and online.	

The condensed skills

		☑ or score (1–5)
Communication skills	Conveying information about genetics in an understandable way; helping patients make informed decisions.	
Consultation skills	Discussing genetic conditions in a non-directive and non-judgemental manner: ● Being aware that people have different attitudes and beliefs about inheritance ● Ensuring your own beliefs do not influence the content of the consultation and the management options offered to a patient.	
History-taking skills	Taking and interpreting a family history (or 'pedigree') to identify patients with, or at risk of, a genetic condition.	

The condensed know-how

	☑ or score (1–5)
The heterogeneity in genetic diseases and understanding the principles of assessing genetic risk, including: ● The principles of risk estimates for family members of patients with Mendelian diseases ● The principles of recurrence risks for simple chromosome anomalies, e.g. trisomies ● How to use online risk assessment tools.	
Local and national referral guidelines and guidelines for managing patients with genetic conditions.	
The organisation of genetics services, where to obtain specialist help and how to make appropriate referrals to genetics services. **Tip:** *There is a national database of genetic centres on the British Society for Human Genetics website: www.bshg.org.uk.*	
The support services available for those with a genetic condition. **Tip:** *Contact a Family offers information on genetic disorders and enables families affected by rare conditions to get in touch with other affected families: www.cafamily.org.uk.*	

	☑ or score (1–5)
The ethical, legal and social implications of genetic information and how it impacts not only on the patient but also on his or her immediate and extended family, and awareness that a genetic diagnosis in an individual may have implications for the management of other family members.	
Issues of confidentiality arising when information about one individual can be used in a predictive manner for another family member.	
The different uses of genetic tests (diagnostic, predictive, carrier testing) and their limitations. **Tip:** *Information on genetic testing can be found at www.ukgtn.nhs.uk and www.genetictestingnetwork.org.uk.*	
The genetic aspects of antenatal and newborn screening programmes (e.g. Down's syndrome, sickle-cell and thalassaemia), and their indications, uses and limitations. **Tip:** *Useful information on the NHS antenatal screening programmes is available at www.screening.nhs.uk/an.*	
Systems for following up patients who have, or are at risk of, a genetic condition and have chosen to undergo regular surveillance. **Tip:** *Does your practice records system have a diary or reminder function?*	
Preventive measures for some genetic conditions. **Tip:** *Familiarise yourself with phenylketonuria (PKU) screening and the Guthrie test (www.newbornscreening-bloodspot.org.uk).*	
The reproductive options available to those with a known genetic condition.	
How the make-up of the local population may affect the prevalence of genetic conditions and attitudes towards genetic disease.	
How a patient's cultural and religious background and beliefs concerning inheritance are important when providing care for people with, or at risk of, genetic conditions. **Tip:** *See condensed statement 3.4:* Promoting Equality and Valuing Diversity.	
The social and psychological impact of a genetic condition on the patient and their family, dependants and employer.	
Awareness that it is not always possible to determine the cause of a condition that may be genetic, or the mutation responsible (e.g. learning disability).	
Ethical and legal issues involved in genetic testing, such as confidentiality, testing children, and pre-symptomatic testing. **Tip:** *Consider the possible implications of genetic testing for obtaining insurance.*	

The condensed resources

- The Primary Care Genetics Society website contains information resources on the management of genetic conditions in primary care: www.pcgs.org.uk.

- NICE has specific guidelines on referral of certain familial conditions for genetic testing (e.g. familial breast cancer): www.nice.org.uk/guidance/cg41.

- British Society for Human Genetics represents genetics professionals: www.bshg.org.uk.

- The NHS National Genetics Education and Development Centre provides education and training in genetics: www.geneticseducation.nhs.uk.

Statement 7: *Care of Acutely Ill People*

Acutely ill people of all ages present unpredictably in general practice, interrupting normal work routines and requiring an urgent response. The effective management of an acutely ill person includes recognition, assessment and immediate management. Organisation, teamwork, communication and situational awareness are also important aspects. A GP must make patient safety a priority and consider the appropriateness of interventions according to a patient's wishes, the severity of the illness and any chronic or co-morbid diseases. GPs must accept responsibility for taking action, at the same time recognising a need to involve more experienced personnel when appropriate, and must keep their resuscitation skills up to date.

Emergency care includes both in-hours and out-of-hours emergencies but particular features of working out of hours, such as isolation, the relative lack of supporting services and the need for proper self-care, require a specific educational focus.

The condensed knowledge

		☑ or score (1–5)
Symptoms	Cardiovascular – chest pain, haemorrhage, shock.	
	Respiratory – wheeze, breathlessness, stridor, choking.	
	Central nervous system – convulsions, reduced conscious level, confusion, unconsciousness.	
	Mental health – threatened self-harm, delusional states, violent patients.	
	Severe pain.	
Conditions	Acute coronary syndromes.	
	Anaphylaxis.	
	Appendicitis.	
	Arrhythmias.	
	Asthma.	
	Bowel obstruction and perforation.	

Continued over

	☑ or score (1–5)

Conditions	Common problems that may be expected with certain practice activities: anaphylaxis after immunisation, local anaesthetic toxicity and vaso-vagal attacks (e.g. during minor surgery or IUD insertion).	
	Dissecting aneurysms.	
	Ectopic pregnancy and antenatal emergencies.	
	Haemorrhage (revealed or concealed).	
	Ischaemia.	
	Malignant hypertension.	
	Meningitis and septicaemia.	
	Parasuicide and suicide attempts.	
	Pulmonary embolus.	
	Pulmonary oedema (severe).	
	Shock (including no cardiac output).	
	Status epilepticus.	
	Understand the principles of managing dangerous diagnoses.	
	Tip: *See table below.*	
Investigation	Blood glucose.	
	Other investigations are rare in primary care because acutely ill patients needing investigation are usually referred to secondary care.	
Treatment	Pre-hospital management of convulsions and acute dyspnoea.	
Emergencies	The 'ABC' principles in initial management.	
	The response time required in order to optimise the outcome for the patient (e.g. 'the golden hour').	
	The organisational aspects of NHS out-of-hours care.	
	Understand the importance of maintaining personal security and awareness and management of the security risks to others.	

		☑ or score (1–5)
Resources	Appropriate use of emergency services, including logistics of how to obtain an ambulance/ paramedic crew.	
	Familiarity with available equipment in own bag/car/practice and that carried by emergency services. **Tip:** *This information should be provided in an induction programme – if not, find out where the emergency equipment is kept and how to use it before an emergency occurs!*	
	Selection and maintenance of the appropriate equipment and un-expired drugs that should be carried by GPs. **Tip:** *There is a useful summary of what to put in a doctor's bag on: www.patient.co.uk/ showdoc/40024568.*	
	Being able to organise and lead a response when required, which may include participation by staff, members of the public or qualified responders.	
	Knowledge of training required for practice staff and others (as a team) in the appropriate responses to an acutely ill person.	
Prevention	Advice to patients on prevention, e.g. with a patient with known heart disease this includes advice on how to manage ischaemic pain, including use of glyceryl trinitrate (GTN), aspirin and appropriate first-line use of paramedic ambulance.	

The condensed skills

		☑ or score (1–5)
Communication skills	Dealing sensitively, and in line with professional codes of practice, with people who may have a serious diagnosis and refuse admission, and presenting a balanced view of the benefits and harms of medical treatment.	

Continued over

		☑ or score (1–5)
Clinical skills	Assessing and managing common medical, surgical and psychiatric emergencies in the in-hours and out-of-hours settings.	
	Tip: *Refer to the emergency sections of each clinical statement in Chapter 7, 'The essential knowledge'.*	
Decision-making skills	Deciding whether or not to admit an acutely ill person and not being unduly influenced by others (such as secondary-care doctors who have not assessed the patient).	
	Tip: *Emergency situations sometimes require more directive approaches to team leadership (e.g. running a resuscitation).*	
Negotiation skills	Dealing with situational crises and manipulative patients, and avoiding the inappropriate use of healthcare resources.	
Psychomotor skills	• Performing and interpreting an ECG.	
	• Cardiopulmonary resuscitation of children and adults including use of a defibrillator.	
	• Controlling a haemorrhage.	
	• Suturing a wound.	
	• Using a nebuliser.	
	• Passing a urinary catheter.	
Risk management skills	Managing personal security and risks to others.	
	Tip: *See condensed statement 3.2:* Patient Safety.	
Stress management skills	Coping with the emotional and stressful aspects of providing acute care.	
Telephone triage skills	Evaluating patient risk, giving advice and making appropriate arrangements to see the patient.	

The condensed know-how

	☑ or score (1–5)

How to recognise, evaluate and manage acutely ill patients, the key differential diagnoses for acutely presenting symptoms.

Tip: *GPs are unlikely to see acutely ill patients with rare conditions very often, which means you may become a bit rusty. Consider keeping easy-to-access protocols in your doctor's bag. Review the Acute Competencies from Foundations Years 1 and 2 (listed in the full curriculum statement 7.)*

Protecting patients with non-urgent and self-limiting problems from being over-investigated, over-treated or deprived of their liberty.

How age, gender, ethnicity, pregnancy, treatment, chronic or co-morbid disease and previous health factors may affect the risk and presentation of acute illness.

Tip: *Always consider ectopic pregnancy as a possible cause of abdominal or pelvic pain in a woman of fertile age.*

How acute illness itself and the anxiety caused by it can impair communication between doctor and patient.

An understanding of local and national protocols, and sources of evidence relating to emergency care and how these may be adapted to unusual circumstances.

Tip: *Resuscitation and other emergency protocols are available from the UK Resuscitation Council (www.resus.org.uk).*

Methods for transporting patients to secondary care and factors to consider when deciding the chosen method and urgency, including when to call 999.

Factors affecting continuity of care in acute illness and steps for minimising problems, including handover and follow-up arrangements.

Tip: *Review the quality of the A&E discharge summaries received by your practice and the issues this raises.*

Factors for deciding in whom resuscitation or intensive care might be inappropriate and how to seek advice on this from carers and colleagues.

Tip: *The Resuscitation Council (www.resus.org.uk) publishes a guideline on 'Do Not Resuscitate' orders.*

How to recognise, confirm, record and certify death, the role of the coroner (or procurator fiscal) and how to provide immediate bereavement support and deal with an unexpected death.

Tip: *Make sure you know what to do if you are called to certify a death at home. This includes providing relevant practical information for the family.*

Continued over

	☑ or score (1–5)
The needs of carers involved at the time of the acutely ill person's presentation and conflicts regarding management that may exist between patients and their relatives.	
Tip: *Consider in which limited situations patient autonomy can be overruled (e.g. mental health emergencies).*	
Ways of recognising and managing patients who are likely to need acute care in the future, and ways to offer them advice on prevention, effective self-management and when and who to call for help.	
Tip: *Find out about case management of those at high risk of admission.*	
Local specialist community resources for acute care or less acute assessment or rehabilitation and how to use these resources appropriately.	
The impact of the doctor's working environment and resources on how acute care is provided.	
Tip: *Make sure you know where your practice keeps emergency equipment and who is responsible for its maintenance and upkeep.*	
The roles of the practice staff in managing acutely ill patients and their relatives.	
Tip: *Do you have a practice protocol in place for dealing with a major incident or flu pandemic?*	
How national NHS emergency and out-of-hours care is organised, and the local arrangements for the provision of out-of-hours care.	
Cultural and other individual factors that might affect emergency management of patients.	
Tip: *Does the patient have specific cultural or religious beliefs that you should take into account (e.g. Jehovah's witness) or a living will?*	
Legal frameworks affecting acute healthcare provision, especially regarding compulsory admission and treatment.	
Tip: *Familiarise yourself with the key sections of the Mental Health Act – GPNotebook has a good summary (www.gpnotebook.co.uk).*	
Patient rights to autonomy and factors that affect an acutely ill patient's capacity for autonomy.	
Tip: *Read up about capacity to consent and the Mental Capacity Act 2005.*	

The condensed resources

- UK resuscitation guidelines can be found on the UK Resuscitation Council website, as well as guidelines on managing anaphylaxis and other emergencies in the community: www.resus.org.uk.

- Doctors.net (www.doctors.net.uk) and RCGP Scotland's PEP eKit (www.pep-ekit.org.uk) contain learning modules on various aspects of emergency care.

- GPNotebook (www.gpnotebook.co.uk) contains clinical information on managing acute medical conditions.

'Dangerous diagnoses'

Research carried out by the Medical Protection Society[24] has identified a number of diagnoses that demand urgent action when the suspicion of them crosses a doctor's mind. Adverse events occur more frequently when a doctor has suspected a potentially dangerous diagnosis but not acted to rule out this possibility. Dangerous diagnoses include:

- Myocardial infarction

- Pulmonary embolus

- Subarachnoid haemorrhage

- Appendicitis

- Limb ischaemia

- Intestinal obstruction or perforation

- Meningitis

- Aneurysms

- Ectopic pregnancy

- Acute psychosis/mania

- Visual problems that could lead to blindness including retinal detachment and haemorrhage as well as systemic disease such as temporal arteritis.

As a general rule, if a GP suspects a dangerous diagnosis is possible, he or she should act as if the diagnosis was certain and refer the patient to the nearest emergency centre. The GP may well be wrong but without having access to appropriate investigations it is far better to be safe than sorry.

Statement 8: *Care of Children and Young People*

Most care for children and young people is delivered outside the hospital setting and there is evidence that good primary care delivers improved health outcomes. A child's experiences in early life have a crucial impact on their life chances. Promoting health can be included in all contacts with a child or young person and their family; this should be targeted particularly at those who are vulnerable or socially excluded.

Safeguarding children and young people requires all GPs to be effective at recognising and dealing with child abuse. GPs should respond to the needs of children and young people in special circumstances, through referral and joint working with relevant services, and should be aware that the needs of young people are different from those of younger children, particularly in terms of their health problems, consent, confidentiality and communication issues.

The condensed knowledge

		☑ or score (1–5)
Symptoms	Abdominal pain (acute and chronic).	
	Behavioural problems.	
	Developmental delay.	
	Failure to thrive and growth disorders.	
	Vomiting, fever, drowsiness.	
Conditions	Bronchiolitis.	
	Child abuse and deprivation.	
	Chronic disease in children: asthma, diabetes, arthritis, learning disability.	
	Constipation.	
	Cough/dyspnoea, wheezing including respiratory infections.	
	Epilepsy.	
	Foreign bodies (e.g. nose, ears, swallowing, inhaling).	
	Gastroenteritis.	

		☑ **or score**
		(1–5)
Conditions	Infant colic.	
	Meningitis.	
	Mental health problems such as attention deficit hyperactivity disorder, depression, eating disorders, substance misuse and self-harm, autistic spectrum disorder and related conditions.	
	Neonatal problems:	
	● Birthmarks	
	● Early feeding problems	
	● Heart murmur	
	● Jaundice	
	● Poor weight gain	
	● Sticky eye.	
	Normal development and developmental problems (physical and psychological).	
	Otitis media.	
	Psychological problems: enuresis, encopresis, bullying, school refusal, behaviour disorders including tantrums.	
	Pyrexia and febrile convulsions.	
	Sensory deficit (especially deafness).	
	Sudden Infant Death Syndrome (SIDS) and strategies to reduce risk.	
	Urinary tract infection.	
	Viral exanthems (childhood illnesses associated with rashes).	
Prevention	Avoiding smoking, using volatile substances and other drugs, and minimising alcohol intake.	
	Breastfeeding.	
	Healthy diet and exercise for children and young people.	
	Immunisation.	

Continued over

		☑ or score (1–5)
Prevention	Keeping children and young people safe: child protection, accident prevention.	
	Prenatal diagnosis.	
	Reducing the risk of teenagers getting pregnant or acquiring sexually transmitted infections.	
	Social and emotional wellbeing.	

The condensed skills

		☑ or score (1–5)
Communication skills	Listening and responding to the sensitivities, health attitudes and behaviours of children and young people, and communicating with parents, carers and families.	
Consultation skills	Enabling children and young people to participate in informed decisions about their care, taking into account their age and development.	
Psychomotor skills	The examination of the newborn child.	
	The six-week check.	
	Basic life support of infants and children.	

The condensed know-how

	☑ or score (1–5)
Safe prescribing in children and young people: ● Calculating drug doses in infants and children ● The risks and benefits of medicines in children and young people. **Tip:** *The BNF for children is a great resource for paediatric prescribing: www.bnfc.org.*	
Information to enable parents or carers, children and young people to manage minor illnesses themselves, to use community pharmacists and triage services, and to access appropriate medical services when necessary. **Tip:** *Patients can obtain free advice on managing minor illness from NHS Direct: www.nhsdirect.nhs.uk.*	

☑ **or score**
(1–5)

Issues around parents with special needs, the role of fathers in parenting, and how to support children of parents with substance misuse, mental health problems or chronic illnesses.

How to promote physical health, mental health and emotional wellbeing, and encourage children, young people and their families to develop healthy lifestyles.

National immunisation programmes and the GP's role in promoting and organising immunisation.

Tip: *This information is contained in the Green Book: www.dh.gov.uk/en/ Policyandguidance/Healthandsocialcaretopics/Greenbook/DH_4097254.*

The GP's role in the prevention of accidents.

Tip: *You can find more information on promoting safety from the Royal Society for the Prevention of Accidents (www.rospa.com).*

Neonatal problems including jaundice and feeding problems, breastfeeding and nutrition.

Normal growth and development of children and young people, and management of delayed development and failure to thrive.

Tip: *Familiarise yourself with the use of growth centile charts and common developmental milestones.*

Problems during transition from child to adolescent, and adolescent to adult, and the effects on the vulnerable or those with chronic diseases.

Tip: *Find out children's and young people's experiences of ill health at www.youthhealthtalk.org.*

How to recognise children and young people at risk, vulnerability factors for children and young people in special circumstances, appropriate referral.

Tip: *All healthcare professionals are required to obtain a Criminal Records Bureau disclosure and to regularly undertake training in child protection.*

The significance of non-attendance:

- Failure to attend can be an indicator of a family's vulnerability, potentially placing the child's welfare in jeopardy

- Acknowledging that failure to attend can be an indicator that services are difficult for families and young people to access or considered inappropriate, and need reviewing.

Tip: *Does your practice have a policy for managing 'DNA's?*

Continued over

☑ or score
(1–5)

Issues around multi-agency working (working across professional and agency boundaries).

Tip: *Familiarise yourself with the issues in this area arising from the Victoria Climbié Inquiry (www.victoria-climbie-inquiry.org.uk).*

Recognising the clinical features of child abuse, knowing about local arrangements for child protection, referring effectively and playing a part in assessment and continuing management (including prevention).

Tip: *Familiarise yourself with your practice's child protection arrangements and where you can find the local child welfare contact details.*

The welfare of the unborn baby and the impact of parental problems including domestic violence, substance misuse and mental health problems, how to recognise such problems (and make a sensitive enquiry) and how to access the relevant local services.

Family, socio-economic and environmental factors, including school, community, ethnicity, cultural issues, inequalities and parenting capacity, that affect health and wellbeing in children and young people.

Issues around design and delivery of services for young people, relating to access, communication, confidentiality and consent.

Tip: *Review the RCGP and RCN joint publication* Getting it Right for Teenagers in Your Practice, *available at: www.rcn.org.uk/members/downloads/getting_it_right.pdf.*

Issues around access for young people to confidential contraceptive and sexual health advice, the design of services tailored to meet their specific needs and the relevant updated guidance.

Tip: *Familiarise yourself with the principles of Gillick/Fraser competency and the best-practice guidance issued by the Department of Health (2004).*[25]

The role of the health visitor and how to undertake a comprehensive child and family needs assessment.

Tip: *Spend a day with a health visitor – they know lots of practical tips and advice on everyday child rearing and behavioural problems.*

The legal and political context and the organisation of child and adolescent care in the NHS, including care pathways and local systems of care.

The impact of childhood disability on the child or young person and their family.

Tip: *Do a case study centred on a child with a disability registered at your practice.*

Recognising inappropriate eating habits such as anorexia nervosa or bulimia and appropriate interventions and services.

Tip: *There are NICE guidelines on eating disorders (www.nice.org.uk).*

The workload issues raised by paediatric problems in the practice, especially the demand for urgent consultations and the mechanisms for dealing with this.

Tip: *Ask the practice manager about 'Advanced Access' appointments systems.*

The issues around treating children and young people equitably and with respect for their beliefs, preferences, dignity and rights (and the relevant legislation), and the issues around confidentiality and consent, record-keeping and sharing information (including legal aspects) relevant to minors.

The condensed resources

- BNF for children: www.bnfc.org.

- Health for all children (Hall 2002): www.healthforallchildren.co.uk.

- Teenager-friendly health advice at www.teenagehealthfreak.org.

- The Royal College of Psychiatrists produces a popular series of leaflets on mental health and behavioural problems in children called *Mental Health and Growing Up*, available at www.rcpsych.ac.uk.

- NICE has guidance on depression in children and young people: www.nice.org.uk.

- SIGN has guidance on bronchiolitis, and the following conditions as they apply to children and young people – epilepsy, obesity, otitis media, attention deficit and hyperkinetic disorders: www.sign.ac.uk.

- Action for Sick Children is a charitable organisation that provides advice and support on children's health issues: www.actionforsickchildren.org.

- The National Service Framework for children sets standards for children's health and social services: www.library.nhs.uk/Default.aspx.

- A key national resource on child protection is www.everychildmatters.gov.uk.

Statement 9: *Care of Older Adults*

The UK has an ageing population and the care of older people will make up an increasing proportion of the GP's workload in the future. Key issues in the care of older people include co-morbidity, difficulties in communicating, the problems of polypharmacy and the need for additional support. GPs have an important role to play in the delivery of improvements in the care of older people, in partnership with the wider primary healthcare team and secondary care.

The condensed skills

		☑ or score (1–5)
Clinical management skills	Managing the concurrent health problems experienced by older people through identification, exploration, negotiation, acceptance and prioritisation.	
Communication skills	Recognising the challenges of communicating with older patients including the slower tempo, possible unreliability of the history and the evidence of third parties.	
Consultation skills	Developing and maintaining a relationship style that treats the older patient with respect and does not patronise.	
Mental health assessment skills	Assessing brain function and mood (e.g. using short mental state questionnaires), and evaluating the testimony of third parties.	

The condensed know-how

	☑ or score (1–5)
The epidemiology of older people's problems in primary care; knowledge of the practice community (e.g. number of elderly patients, prevalence of chronic diseases).	
The theories of ageing; the physical (including lab values), psychological and social changes that occur with age and relating them to the adaptations that an older person makes, and to the breakdown of these adaptations.	

or score
(1–5)

The effect of physical factors, particularly diet, exercise temperature and sleep, on the health of older people and the interrelationships between health and social care.

The concept of co-morbidity.

Features relating to prognosis of diseases in old age and how this informs an appropriate plan for further investigation and management.

The management of the conditions and problems commonly associated with old age such as Parkinson's disease, falls, gait disorders, stroke and confusion.

Tip: *The Royal College of Physicians produces guidance in this area, available at www.rcplondon.ac.uk/specialty/Geriatric.asp.*

Drug treatment in the elderly, the physiology of absorption, metabolism and excretion of drugs, the hazards posed by multiple prescribing, non-compliance and iatrogenic disease, the importance of medication reviews and the issue of medication errors and iatrogenic disease.

Tip: *Review the concept of polypharmacy and the Beers criteria[26] (medication inappropriate for elderly people); the BNF has a section on prescribing in the elderly.*

Issues around access to the primary healthcare team for older people, including geographical distance, appropriate timing of appointments and the organisational approach to the management of chronic conditions and co-morbidities.

Knowledge of the locally agreed protocols for preventing and managing health problems in the elderly (e.g. stroke).

Tip: *The Royal College of Physicians (www.rcplondon.ac.uk) has produced guidelines on the management of stroke.*

Issues around the transfer from one system of care to another, the complications that can arise and how they can be prevented and managed.

Tip: *Consider spending time with a local geriatrician and find out what specialist services are available in your area. Do you have a falls clinic or geriatric day hospital?*

Support services for older patients (e.g. podiatry, visual and hearing aids, immobility and walking aids, meals on wheels, home care services), different forms of day care and residential accommodation, and the various statutory and voluntary organisations for older people in the community.

Tip: *District nurses are often excellent sources of this information.*

Continued over

Quality assurance of elderly care, including policies on repeat prescriptions, the appropriate use of screening and case-finding programmes, and auditing the quality of care.

Tip: *Review your practice's repeat prescribing policy and the procedure for medication reviews.*

How the provision of care can affect the patient's sense of identity and dignity, and ways of ensuring patients are not discriminated against due to their age, and the issues of recognising and dealing with elder abuse.

The legal issues relevant to the elderly including confidentiality, Mental Health Act, power of attorney, court of protection, guardianship, living wills, death certification and cremation.

Tip: *Have a tutorial on the paperwork related to death, in particular when it is necessary to involve the police or the coroner.*

The special features of psychiatric diseases in old age, the features of dementia, and the effects of physical function on the mental state.

Ethical tensions between the needs of the elderly individual and the community.

Tip: *Consider the ethical problems raised when advising an elderly patient on his or her fitness to drive and the DVLA regulations.*

How preventive strategies can be adapted to older people.

Tip: *Look into strategies for preventing falls in the elderly.*

The key government policy documents, national guidelines and research findings that influence healthcare provision for older people.

Tip: *The NSF for older people can be found at: www.library.nhs.uk/Default.aspx.*

The condensed resources

- NICE (www.nice.org.uk) has clinical guidelines on dementia.

- SIGN (www.sign.ac.uk) has guidelines on the prevention and management of hip fracture in older people.

- DVLA guidelines can be found at www.dvla.gov.uk/medical/ataglance.aspx.

- Age Concern offers information and support for the elderly on health and social care: www.ace.org.uk.

- The British Geriatrics Society is the professional body for specialists in old-age medicine and psychiatry of old age: www.bgs.org.uk.

- The National Service Framework for older people (www.library.nhs.uk) sets out the standards for the care of older people as does its Scottish equivalent *Adding Life to Years* (2001):[27] www.scotland.gov.uk/library3/health/alty-00.asp.

Statement 10.1: *Women's Health*

Women's health issues, including contraception, pregnancy, menopause and disorders of the reproductive organs, account for over 25 per cent of how a GP spends his or her time. In society, women tend to play a larger role in caring for dependent relatives and children, and GPs play an important part in supporting women in this role. GPs are also responsible for diagnosing domestic violence and dealing with its physical and psychological effects.

The condensed knowledge

		☑ or score (1–5)
Symptoms	Breast pain, breast lumps, nipple discharge.	
	Dyspareunia, pelvic pain, endometriosis.	
	Emotional problems, including low mood and symptoms of depression.	
	Faecal incontinence.	
	Infertility – primary and secondary.	
	Menopause and menopausal problems.	
	Period-related problems.	
	Post-menopausal bleeding.	
	Pruritus vulvae, vaginal discharge.	
	Urinary malfunction: dysuria, frequency, incontinence.	
Conditions	Abnormal cervical cytology.	
	Fibroids.	
	Gynaecological infections, including Bartholin's abscess.	
	Gynaecological malignancies.	
	Intrauterine infection.	
	Menstrual disorders:	
	• Amenorrhoea	
	• Dysmenorrhoea	

		☑ **or score**
		(1–5)

Conditions	● Inter-menstrual bleeding	
	● Menorrhagia	
	● Pre-menstrual syndrome.	
	Mental health issues specific to women including anxiety, depression, parasuicide, eating disorders, self-harming and the relationship between these, pregnancy and the menopause.	
	Pregnancy (including normal antenatal and postnatal care):	
	Tip: *Spend a day on attachment with the community midwife.*	
	● Abnormal lies and placenta praevia	
	● Anaemia	
	● Antepartum haemorrhage and abruption	
	● Common problems including hyperemesis, acid reflux, back pain, symphysis pubis dysfunction, leg ache and varicose veins and haemorrhoids	
	● Deep-vein thrombosis and pulmonary embolism, post dates, reduced movements	
	● Ectopic pregnancy	
	● Gestational diabetes	
	● Growth retardation	
	● Intrauterine death and foetal abnormality	
	● Miscarriage and abortion	
	● Multiple pregnancy	
	● Poly- and oligohydramnios	
	● Pre-eclampsia and hypertension in pregnancy	
	● Premature labour	
	● Rhesus status and role of anti-D	
	● Trophoblastic disease.	
	Sexual dysfunction including psychosexual conditions.	
	Vaginal and uterine prolapse.	

Continued over

		☑ or score (1–5)
Investigation	Pregnancy testing.	
	Urinalysis, MSU (mid-stream specimen of urine) and urine dipstick.	
	Blood tests including renal function tests, hormone tests.	
	Bacteriological and virology tests.	
	Knowledge of secondary-care investigations including colposcopy and subfertility investigations.	
Treatment	Primary-care management of the conditions listed above.	
	Menopause management including the pros and cons of hormone replacement therapy (HRT).	
	Knowledge of specialist treatments and surgical procedures including: laparoscopy, D&C (dilation and curettage), hysterectomy, oophorectomy, ovarian cystectomy, pelvic floor repair, medical and surgical termination of pregnancy, sterilisation.	
	Understand the risks of prescribing during pregnancy.	
Emergencies	Bleeding in pregnancy.	
	Suspected ectopic pregnancy.	
	Domestic violence.	
Prevention	Health education regarding lifestyle and sexual and mental health.	
	Pre-pregnancy issues discontinuing contraception, folic acid, family and genetic history, and lifestyle advice.	
	Pregnancy care including health promotion, social and cultural factors, smoking and alcohol, diet, age factors and previous obstetric history.	
	Rubella testing and immunisation.	
	Risk assessment, screening and management of osteoporosis.	

The condensed skills

		☑ or score (1–5)
Communication skills	Talking sensitively with women about sexuality and intimate issues.	
Psychomotor skills	Breast examination.	
Tip: *Always pay attention to professional etiquette, providing information, obtaining informed consent and ensuring patient comfort.*	Catheterisation.	
	Cervical smear.	
	Changing a ring pessary.	
	Pelvic examination (including digital and speculum examination, assessment of the size, position and mobility of the uterus, and the recognition of abnormality of the pelvic organs).	
	Use of sonicaid/foetal stethoscope.	
Self-awareness and reflective skills	Identifying own values, attitudes and approach to ethical issues (e.g. abortion, contraception for minors, consent, confidentiality, cosmetic surgery).	

The condensed know-how

	☑ or score (1–5)
Primary-care management of women's risk factors, health problems, conditions and diseases. **Tip:** *Consider completing the course to obtain the Diploma of the Royal College of Obstetricians and Gynaecologists, especially if you have a secondary-care O&G post in your training programme.*	
The indications for urgent referral to specialist services, for patients with breast lumps, gynaecological or obstetric emergencies. **Tip:** *Find out how to obtain urgent early pregnancy scans and assessment.*	
Screening strategies relevant to women (e.g. cervical, breast, other cancers, postnatal depression) and their advantages/disadvantages, and tensions between the science and politics of screening. **Tip:** *Review the Edinburgh Postnatal Depression Scale.*	
Prevention strategies relevant to women (e.g. safer sex, pre-pregnancy counselling, antenatal care, immunisation, osteoporosis) and issues around health promotion, and the impact of this on the unborn child, growing children and the family.	

Continued over

Awareness of local support services, referral services, networks and groups for women.

Tip: *Familiarise yourself with local family planning services, breast cancer nurses and domestic violence resources.*

The key national guidelines that influence women's healthcare provision.

The issues around equity and access to information and health services for women, practice management issues affecting the provision of care to women including availability of female doctors and informing patients of results of screening and ensuring follow-up, and the role of well-woman clinics.

Tip: *Evaluate the effectiveness of the primary-care service you provide from the female patient's point of view.*

The prevalence of domestic violence and question sensitively where this may be an issue.

Tip: *This is covered in the full curriculum statement 10.1*: Women's Health.

Confidentiality issues that relate to women (family issues, domestic violence, termination of pregnancy, sexually transmitted infections and 'Partner Notification').

The issues relating to the use of chaperones in women's healthcare.

Tip: *Find out what arrangements your practice has for providing chaperones.*

The issues of gender and power, and the effect of this on the doctor–patient relationship.

The impact of gender on individual cognition and lifestyle, and strategies for responding to this.

The impact of culture and ethnicity on women's perceived role in society and their attendant health beliefs, and how to tailor health care accordingly.

The psycho-social component of women's health and the need, in some cases, to provide women patients with additional emotional and organisational support (e.g. in relation to pregnancy options, hormone replacement therapy, breast cancer and unemployment).

Legislation relevant to women's health (e.g. abortion, contraception).

Tip: *Familiarise yourself with the criteria relating to termination on the 'blue form' (Certificate A).*

The condensed resources

- NICE (www.nice.org.uk) has issued clinical guidelines on long-acting reversible contraception, fertility, antenatal care, postnatal care, heavy menstrual bleeding, and urinary incontinence. It has also issued technology appraisals on cervical screening.

- SIGN (www.sign.ac.uk) has guidance on investigation of postmenopausal bleeding, postnatal depression and puerperal psychosis, breast cancer and osteoporosis.

- The Royal College of Obstetricians and Gynaecologists has issued a number of relevant guidelines: www.rcog.org.uk.

- The National Screening Committee (www.nsc.nhs.uk) website contains guidelines on screening for breast, cervical and ovarian cancer.

Statement 10.2: *Men's Health*

Overall, men suffer more ill health than women and their life expectancy is five years lower. Men tend to take more risks with their health and have higher rates of alcohol misuse, smoking, poor diet, sexually transmitted diseases and accidents. Consultation rates are lower in men than women, and these rates have declined further in recent years. Men also have a higher risk of committing suicide compared with women.

The condensed knowledge

		☑ or score (1–5)
Symptoms	Abdominal and loin pains.	
	Erectile dysfunction.	
	Haematuria.	
	Retention of urine.	
	Sore/painful penis, ulceration, skin changes.	
	Testicular lumps.	
	Testicular pain (orchalgia).	
	Urinary symptoms: dysuria, frequency, nocturia, poor stream, prostatism.	
Conditions	Benign prostatic hypertrophy (BPH) and prostatitis.	
	Circumcision (religious and non-religious).	
	Male contraception: vasectomy.	
	Male infertility.	
	Male-specific cancers: testicular and prostate cancer.	
	Mental health issues including depression, suicide and andropause.	
	Other testicular conditions, e.g. cryptorchidism, varicocele, haematocele, hydrocele, epididymo-orchitis and epidydmitis.	
	Sexual dysfunction including psychosexual conditions, premature ejaculation and erectile dysfunction.	

		☑ or score (1–5)
Investigation	Urinalysis, MSU and dipstick.	
	Blood tests including renal function tests and prostate-specific antigen (PSA) test.	
	Semen analysis.	
	Knowledge of secondary-care investigations including prostate biopsy and testicular ultrasound.	
Treatment	Understand principles of treatment for common conditions managed largely in primary care – benign prostatic hypertrophy, prostatitis, sexual dysfunction, infertility, etc.	
	Injection of anti-androgens for testicular cancer.	
Emergencies	Acute management of testicular torsion.	
	Acute management of paraphimosis and priapism	
	Acute urinary retention.	
	Acute management of ureteric colic.	
Prevention	Health education regarding lifestyle and risk-taking behaviour, sexual and mental health.	

The condensed skills

		☑ or score (1–5)
Communication skills	Developing a non-judgemental, caring and professional consulting style to minimise any embarrassment.	
	Compensating, when necessary, for men being less articulate about their health.	
	Encouraging men to express and modify their health beliefs.	

Continued over

	☑ or score (1–5)
Psychomotor skills	Testicular examination.	
Tip: *Always pay attention to professional etiquette, providing information, obtaining informed consent and ensuring patient comfort.*	Digital rectal examination.	
	Catheterisation.	
	Injection/implantation of anti-androgens for testicular cancer.	
Risk management	Understanding that violence and aggression are more common amongst young men, how to assess the risk of harm to the patient, yourself and others, and intervene appropriately.	

The condensed know-how

	☑ or score (1–5)
Primary-care management of men's risk factors, health problems, conditions and diseases (and the relative prevalence of medical conditions in men compared with women), including care of men with genito-urinary problems.	
The indications for urgent referral to specialist services, for patients with emergencies including testicular lumps and suspected testicular cancer. **Tip:** *Review the NICE referral for suspected cancer guidelines.*	
Men's consulting patterns. **Tip:** *Consider how your surgery appointments system and the limited availability of late or weekend surgeries affects men's access to health care.*	
The psychological, social, cultural and economic problems caused by unemployment amongst men, local demography, social deprivation and service provision factors that may contribute to poor male health.	
How relationships with male patients will differ depending on the gender of the doctor, and how and when to intervene when this is adversely affecting the doctor–patient relationship.	
The impact of gender on individual cognitions and lifestyle, and strategies for responding to this, and the changing gender roles to which men are expected to conform.	

☑ or score
(1–5)

How cultural background may affect a man's attitudes towards health and expectations of the doctor.	
The particular difficulties that adolescent males have when accessing primary-care services. **Tip:** *Read the BMA report (December 2003) on adolescent care here: www.bma.org.uk/ap.nsf/Content/AdolescentHealth.*	
Screening strategies relevant to men, the indications for a PSA blood test, its role in the diagnosis and management of prostate cancer, the arguments for and against a national PSA screening programme. **Tip:** *www.cancerscreening.nhs.uk/prostate/informationpack.html has useful information, including patient information leaflets, on PSA screening.*	
Health promotion and disease prevention strategies (e.g. safe sex) for men and techniques for opportunistic health education during consultations with infrequent attenders. **Tip:** *Consider the role of the practice nurse in delivering effective health promotion for men.*	
The impact of illness, in both the male patient and his family, on the presentation and management, and of men's health problems. **Tip:** *Self-employed people may not receive much sick pay when they are ill.*	
The features of a successful men's health service, practical means of engaging with men more effectively, the role of well-man clinics in primary care. **Tip:** *Evaluate the effectiveness of the primary-care service you provide from the male patient's point of view.*	

The condensed resources

Understanding men's health involves three main themes:[28]

1. Biological determinants
2. Lifestyle and individual risk taking
3. Masculinity and socialisation.

- The evidence-based journal Bandolier has an interesting men's health collection: www.jr2.ox.ac.uk/bandolier/booth/booths/men.html.

- The Men's Health Forum (www.menshealthforum.org.uk) promotes men's health policy development and runs a site providing health advice aimed at men: www.malehealth.co.uk.

- The International Society for Men's Health and Gender provides relevant publications and a forum for exchanging information on men's health issues: www.ismh.org.

- The website www.embarrassingproblems.co.uk is a useful resource to direct embarrassed teenagers (and adults!).

Statement 11: *Sexual Health*

GPs have an important role in the management of sexual health problems, including sexually transmitted infections (STIs) and sexual dysfunction, in partnership with other members of the primary healthcare team and specialists. Primary healthcare teams are ideally placed to take a holistic and integrated approach to sexual health, which is a UK health priority. GP education should promote integrated learning about sexual health within the complex team of the NHS.

The condensed knowledge

		☑ or score (1–5)
Symptoms	Abnormal genital smell.	
	Ano-genital lumps.	
	Genital skin conditions including rashes, ulcers and lichen sclerosis.	
	Intermenstrual bleeding.	
	Lower abdominal pain in women.	
	Pain on intercourse.	
	Pain on passing urine in men and women.	
	Testicular pain and swelling.	
	Unusual or different vaginal discharge or penile urethral discharge.	
	Vaginal bleeding after sex.	
Conditions	Ano-genital ulcers – herpes simplex, syphilis, tropical infections, primary HIV infection.	
	Ano-genital warts.	
	Bacterial vaginosis.	
	Candidiasis.	
	Chlamydial infections.	
	Conditions suggestive of immunosuppression (e.g. pneumocystis, pneumonia, tuberculosis, lymphoma, seborrhoeic dermatitis or oral thrush) or of primary HIV infection.	

Continued over

		☑ or score (1–5)

Conditions	Conjunctivitis (neonatal and adult).	
	Gonorrhoea.	
	Group B haemolytic streptococcus. **Tip:** *Familiarise yourself with your local protocol on antenatal screening for Group B strep.*	
	HIV and AIDS and the presentations/complications including pneumocystis pneumonia, candidiasis, cryptococcus, Kaposi's sarcoma, toxoplasmosis, lymphoma, hepatitis, tuberculosis.	
	Reiter's syndrome.	
	Sexual dysfunction.	
	Sexual identity disorders and gender realignment.	
	Syphilis.	
	Trichomonas vaginalis.	
Investigation	Pregnancy testing.	
	Urinalysis, MSU and dipstick.	
	Approaches to the diagnosis of bacterial vaginosis.	
	Blood tests for HIV and appropriate counselling.	
	Blood tests for syphilis and their interpretation.	
	Blood tests for hepatitis B and their interpretation.	
	Microbiology and virology swabs – which to use, which samples to take, limitations of tests and interpretation of results.	
	Secondary-care investigations, e.g. colposcopy.	
Treatment	Contraception – effectiveness rates, risks, benefits and appropriate selection of patients for all methods, including methods of emergency contraception.	
	Contraception – the safe provision of all methods of oral contraception (including emergency hormonal contraception) and also contraceptive patches and DMPA injections.	

		☑ or score (1–5)
Treatment	Contraception – knowledge and availability of intrauterine methods of contraception (including as a method of emergency contraception), subdermal implants, sterilisation and natural family planning.	
	Abortion – methods and the legal procedures relating to referral for abortion. **Tip:** *Find out the local arrangements for women requesting termination of pregnancy.*	
	Principles of treatment for common conditions diagnosed and/or managed in primary care (see above).	
	Principles of antiretroviral combination therapy for HIV/AIDS, potential side effects and the role of the GP in their management in primary care.	
Prevention	Emergency hormonal contraception.	

The condensed skills

		☑ or score (1–5)
Counselling skills	Counselling patients with sexual problems including psychosexual issues related to contraception, sexually transmitted infection, HIV testing, and for patients who have an unplanned or unwanted pregnancy.	
Psychomotor skills **Tip:** *Always pay attention to professional etiquette, providing information, obtaining informed consent and ensuring patient comfort.*	Performing a sexual health examination including digital and speculum examination.	
	Intramuscular injection.	
	Taking microbiology and virology swabs from ano-genital areas.	
	Teaching the patient about male and female condom use.	
	Injection/implantation of anti-androgens for testicular cancer.	

Continued over

		☑ or score (1–5)
Risk assessment skills	Tailoring advice and care accordingly, including advice on safer sexual practices and hepatitis B immunisation.	
Self-awareness and reflective skills	Ensuring that your own beliefs, or moral or religious reservations, about any contraceptive methods, abortion or sexual behaviours do not adversely affect the management of a patient's sexual health.	
Sexual history-taking skills **Tip:** *Attending a STIF course is a good way to practise these skills: www.bashh.org.*	Taking a sexual history from a male or female patient (in a way that is confidential, non-judgemental, responsive to the patient and avoids assumptions about sexual orientation or the gender of the partner, or assumptions related to age, disability or ethnic origin).	
	Using sexual history (including partner history and information on sexual practices including condom use) and other relevant information to assess risk of STI, unwanted pregnancy and cervical cancer.	
	Applying the information gathered to generate a differential diagnosis and formulate a management plan.	

The condensed know-how

	☑ or score (1–5)
The epidemiology of sexual health problems and how this is reflected in the local population. **Tip:** *Consider the sexual health needs of specific populations (e.g. students).*	
Factors affecting accessibility of sexual health services and strategies to improve this.	
Referral criteria to local specialist services, including gynaecologists, sexual and reproductive health specialists, genito-urinary specialists, urologists, specialists in infectious diseases and specialists in sexual dysfunction.	

☑ **or score**
(1–5)

Strategies for the promotion of sexual health and the early detection of sexual health problems that may have not yet produced symptoms.	
Tip: *Does your practice offer chlamydia screening?*	
Confidentiality issues related to sexual health.	
Tip: *Find out about the doctor's duty of confidentiality and the issues raised by the Sexual Offences Act 2003 (different guidance applies in different countries in the UK).*	
The functional anatomy of the male and female genital systems, and the female reproductive physiology.	
Common presentations of sexual dysfunction, and of sexual violence and abuse, including covert presentations such as somatisation.	
When urgent intervention and referral is needed appropriately, e.g. in provision of emergency contraception or in severe pelvic inflammatory disease, or in serious infections in the immune-compromised patient.	
The limitations of 'watching and waiting' because some serious infections (e.g. chlamydia and HIV) may lapse back into being asymptomatic whilst causing harm to the patient.	
Risk factors for cervical cancer and the value of an opportunistic approach to screening in this group.	
Cervical smear abnormalities, referral criteria, and what is involved in secondary-care management.	
Tip: *Arrange a clinical attachment at your local colposcopy department.*	
Specific interventions for HIV prevention such as post-exposure prophylaxis and the prevention of mother-to-baby transmission.	
Sexual health screening programmes in use in the UK and the benefits, limitations and need for informed consent.	
Tip: *See condensed statement 5:* Healthy People *for more information on the issues around screening.*	
Patient groups at greater risk of unplanned pregnancies and value of opportunistic approach for health promotion and contraception advice, and the role of GPs and primary care teams in the prevention of unwanted pregnancies.	
Principles of and current guidance for partner notification.	

Continued over

How to access local sexual health services, including services that provide specialist contraceptive care; termination of pregnancy; STI diagnosis and management; HIV management and services for relationship problems and sexual dysfunction.

TIP: *Consider spending a session attached to your local sexual health clinic.*

Cultural and existential factors that affect the patient's risk of having sexual health problems and also his or her reactions to them, and the social stigma often associated with sexual health problems or sexual orientation/behaviour, even in some healthcare professionals.

Factors associated with risky sexual behaviour including mental health problems, drug and alcohol misuse, and a history of sexual abuse, and the wider determinants of unplanned pregnancies and their impact on the individual and society.

Patient groups where sexual health consideration may be inappropriately omitted by health professionals (those with physical or learning disabilities or the elderly).

Legal aspects relating to sexual health including termination of pregnancy and the methods used in the UK, and the provision of contraception and sexual health treatment in under-16s (including child protection).

Tip: *Aspects include the Fraser guidelines relating to the Gillick case, the Human Rights Act 1998 and the Sexual Offences Act 2003.*

Ethical principles involved when treating patients who have sexual health concerns (e.g. contraception and abortion).

Key national guidelines that influence sexual healthcare provision.

The condensed resources

- The course for the Diploma of the Faculty of Family Planning and Reproductive Healthcare (www.ffprhc.org.uk) is a solid foundation for learning about the management of sexual health problems.

- NICE (www.nice.org.uk) has guidance on long-acting reversible contraception, and fertility.

- SIGN (www.sign.ac.uk) has guidance on management of chlamydia infection.

- The FPA has information on contraception and sexually transmitted infections: www.fpa.org.uk/information/leaflets.

- The British Association for Sexual Health and HIV: www.bashh.org.

- The Terrence Higgins Trust provides a wide range of publications and information on HIV, AIDS and sexual health for health professionals and the public: www.tht.org.uk.

- Relate offers a psychosexual counselling service in addition to its relationship counselling services: www.relate.org.uk.

Statement 12: *Care of People with Cancer and Palliative Care*

In the curriculum, 'cancer' is considered as a generic term rather than a set of site-specific diseases (individual conditions are covered in the relevant statements). The GP's role extends from primary prevention of cancer through early diagnosis to palliation and terminal care. Cancer is a concern for many patients who consult their doctor and one of the great skills of a good GP is to recognise cancer in its early stages.

GPs are responsible for the palliative care of both cancer and non-cancer patients. Enabling patients to die with dignity and with minimal distress is one of the most fundamental aspects of medicine. Many terminally ill patients prefer the option of a death at home and the primary-care team has a crucial role to play in managing this process.

The condensed knowledge

		☑ or score (1–5)
Emergencies	Anxiety/panic.	
	Hypercalcaemia.	
	Major haemorrhage.	
	Pancytopenia.	
	Pathological bone fractures.	
	Spinal cord compression.	
	Superior vena caval obstruction.	
Treatment	Knowledge about a syringe driver:	
	• Suitable drugs	
	• Conversion of drugs from oral dosage to syringe drive, either IV or subcutaneous.	
	Tip: *Read the BNF section on 'Prescribing in Palliative Care'.*	
	Use of emergency drugs in palliative care.	

The condensed skills

		☑ or score (1–5)
Clinical skills	Attending to the full range of physical, psychological, social and spiritual needs of the patient and carers.	
Communication skills	Communicating sensitively and effectively with the patient and carer(s) regarding difficult information about the disease, its treatment or its prognosis.	
Counselling skills	Advising, motivating and explaining: • Risk of disease • Behaviour change • Treatment options • Symptom control.	
Leadership and team-working skills	Functioning both as leader and member of cancer care teams as required.	
Psychomotor skills	Setting up a syringe driver.	
Reflective and housekeeping skills	Addressing your personal attitudes and experiences that can affect your attitude towards patients with cancer or who are dying.	

The condensed know-how

	☑ or score (1–5)
The epidemiology of major cancers along with risk factors and unhealthy behaviours, current population trends in the prevalence of risk factors and cancer in the community, and how geographical factors influence the prevalence and treatment of cancers.	
The principles and design of primary and secondary cancer screening programmes. **Tip:** *See condensed statement 5: Healthy People.*	
Signs and symptoms of the early presentation of cancer and the appropriate investigations of patients with suspected cancer, including referral guidelines and protocols (local and national). **Tip:** *NICE has issued clinical guidelines for GPs on the referral of patients with suspected cancer.*	

Continued over

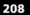

☑ **or score**
(1–5)

The principles of palliative care and how they apply to non-cancer illnesses such as cardiovascular, neurological, respiratory and infectious diseases.

Tip: *Remember this includes the palliative care of children.*

Factors affecting the provision of 24-hour continuity of care through various clinical systems.

Tip: *Find out how to notify your local out-of-hours service about palliative and terminally ill patients.*

Pain management (assessing and treating pain).

Tip: *Learn the WHO pain relief ladder: www.who.int/cancer/palliative/painladder.*

The social benefits and services available to patients and carers.

Tip: *Find out the rules on the DS1500 form for claiming benefits for the terminally ill.*

The social and psychological impact of cancer on the patient's family, friends, dependants and employers.

Tip: *Find out how to arrange respite care or overnight nursing.*

The normal and abnormal grieving process and its impact upon symptomatology.

Tip: *Well-recognised bereavement models include the phases of grief, tasks of mourning, dimensions of loss and dual process.*

The key health service policy documents that influence provision for cancer and palliative care.

Ethical and legal dimensions of treatment and investigation choices, palliative and terminal care, euthanasia and advanced directives.

Tip: *The Dignity in Dying charity (formerly the Voluntary Euthanasia Society) provides information on living wills: www.dignityindying.org.uk.*

Cancer treatment trials and the issues around patient participation in trials.

The condensed resources

- SIGN (www.sign.ac.uk) has guidelines on the control of pain in patients with cancer.

- The Palliative Care Gold Standards can be accessed at www.goldstandardsframework.nhs.uk.

- NHS Cancer Screening Programme: www.cancerscreening.nhs.uk.

- See the example learning plan for this statement illustrated in Table 3.5 in Chapter 3, 'Learning the curriculum'.

- Macmillan Cancer Support offers support to patients with cancer and produces advice leaflets: www.macmillan.co.uk.

- Marie Curie Cancer Care provides free nursing care to terminally ill people to give them the choice of dying at home: www.mariecurie.org.uk.

- Cancer Research UK provides news, statistics and information on cancer: www.cancerresearchuk.org.

- Cruse Bereavement Care offers advice on the normal bereavement process and provides counselling and support to people who have been bereaved: www.crusebereavementcare.org.uk.

Statement 13: *Care of People with Mental Health Problems*

Providing care for people with mental health problems is integral to the work of a GP, represents a significant workload and has implications for the public health of the practice population. Mental health problems seen in primary care include a large range of conditions. In particular, GPs should be able to recognise depression and assess its severity; all depressed patients should be screened for suicidal intent. People with severe mental illness have a high prevalence of physical co-morbidity that must also be managed.

GPs should be aware that all physical illness has a psychological component; this should be taken into account in management plans. Developing skills to recognise and manage somatisation could lead to considerable savings in both terms of patient suffering and healthcare costs. Continuous improvement of communication skills and patient-centred practice is likely to be the single most important factor in improving the recognition and effective management of mental health problems.

The condensed knowledge

		☑ or score (1–5)
Symptoms	Abdominal pain and bowel upset (i.e. somatisation).	
	Anxiety.	
	Depression.	
	Dizziness, palpitations and paraesthesiae.	
	Early signs of possible psychotic illness.	
	Insomnia.	
	Multiple somatic complaints.	
	Tired all the time (when physical causes excluded).	
Conditions	Attention deficit hyperactivity disorder (ADHD).	
	Alcohol and drug misuse (see condensed statement 15.3).	
	Anxiety disorders.	
	Depression.	

		☑ or score (1–5)
Conditions	Eating disorders.	
	Personality disorder.	
	Post-traumatic stress disorder.	
	Schizophrenia and psychotic illness.	
	Somatisation disorder.	
Investigation	Use of depression rating scales, and other aids to evaluation of possible diagnosis and severity.	
Treatment	Pharmacology.	
	CBT and simple behavioural techniques.	
	Problem-solving therapy.	
	Basis of systemic and strength-focused therapies.	
	Self-administered therapy.	
Emergencies	Threatened or attempted suicide.	
	Delirium.	
	Psychosis.	
	Panic.	
	Aggressive or violent patients.	
	Drug overdose and alcohol withdrawal.	
Resources	The family of the patient.	
	Members of the primary healthcare team, receptionist, counsellor, Citizens Advice Bureau (CAB) worker.	
	Specialist mental health services and non-medical agencies (non-professional, lay or voluntary resources).	
Prevention	Mental health promotion, especially children, families and adolescents.	
	Screening of all language-delayed children for autism.	
	Early intervention in psychosis.	

The condensed skills

		☑ or score (1–5)
Consultation skills	Establishing rapport with the patient and family.	
	Integrating physical, psychological and social ideas.	
	Avoiding medicalising common mental distresses and dealing appropriately with the uncertainty that certain patients may produce.	
	Responding quickly and appropriately to concerns raised by relatives and others.	
Psychomotor skills	Mental state assessment.	
	Suicide risk assessment.	
Self-awareness and reflective skills	Self-awareness and reflective skills (to develop a personal management plan for your own mental health and to understand how your own attitudes and feelings affect how you manage): • People who self-harm • People who misuse drugs or alcohol • People who know more about their illnesses than their doctors do • People who engender strong emotions.	

The condensed know-how

	☑ or score (1–5)
Risk factors for mental health problems, the difference between depression and emotional distress, how to identify mental health problems that are covert or somatised. **Tip:** *Risk factors are described in Appendix 7 of the full curriculum statement.*	
Diagnostic criteria for people experiencing mental health problems. **Tip:** *Familiarise yourself with DSM and ICD systems for classifying mental health disorders.*	

	☑ or score (1–5)

How to screen for mental illness, using effective and reliable instruments, and issues around the screening and diagnosis of people with physical illness.

Tip: *Find out about screening tools (e.g. 'two questions'[29]) and diagnostic questionnaires used in your practice (examples include HAD and PHQ-9 – see the condensed resources).*

Management of mental health problems in primary care, including different forms of talking therapy, medication and self-help.

Tip: *Find out about common forms of talking treatment (counselling, problem solving, CBT, psychodynamic psychotherapy, supportive counselling).*

Specific interventions and guidelines for individual mental health conditions, as described in the SIGN or NICE guidelines and stepped models of intervention.

Early indicators of psychological difficulties in children and young people, and ways that a first episode of psychosis may present in the young.

Issues around frequent attenders, patients who demand drugs, and chronic suicidicity in borderline personality disorder.

Tip: *Discuss various strategies for dealing with demanding patients in your learning group – there are no easy answers.*

Psychosomatic complaints, psychological consequences of physical illness and somatisation.

How to access mental health and social care organisations, both voluntary and statutory.

Tip: *Find out about the local mental health service arrangements in your area, especially the phone numbers of the local mental health crisis teams and who to refer to 'out of hours' (often after 5 p.m.).*

When is it appropriate to refer to and collaborate with the specialist mental health services?

Tip: *See Appendix 6 of the full curriculum statement for more information.*

Responsibilities for supporting children in difficulty and how to access support and advice from specialist child and adolescent mental health workers in primary care.

The concept of concordance; how it is particularly important in mental health care and how presenting individuals with choices can improve the effectiveness of intervention.

Continued over

☑ or score
(1–5)

The particular issues around continuity of care for people with mental health problems.

Tip: *Find out about the Care Programme Approach (CPA) and the role of the key worker or care coordinator.*

The prevalence of mental health problems and needs amongst the practice population and any relevant local health improvement programmes.

The associated physical health problems of people with mental health problems.

Tip: *Particular problems involve lifestyle issues including smoking, drug misuse, weight disorders and difficulties using health services appropriately.*

The principles of mental health promotion (see Appendix 5).

The impact of social circumstances on mental illness and recovery, and the principles of promoting recovery (see Appendix 8).

The extent and implications of stigma and social exclusion relating to mental illness.

Tip: *You can learn about patients' own experiences of living with mental illness at: www.dipex.org.*

Cultural determinants of mental illness and the problems caused by assumptions that may not be universally held.

The use of value judgements in psychiatric diagnosis and the concept of a values-based approach to mental health.

Ethical issues around compulsory treatment and the use of psychotropic drugs to sedate people for social reasons, and the role of drug companies in promoting psychotropic drugs.

Sufficient knowledge of the current Mental Health Act and the responsibilities of a GP.

Tip: *Learn about the role of the approved social worker and try to observe a Mental Health Act assessment at least once during your training.*

The condensed resources

- NSF on mental health: www.library.nhs.uk.

- NICE (www.nice.org.uk) has clinical guidelines on anxiety, bipolar disorder, dementia, depression, depression in children and young people, eating disorders, obsessive-compulsive disorder, post-traumatic stress disorder, schizophrenia, self-harm and violence. It has also commissioned technology appraisals on atypical antipsychotics, newer hypnotic drugs for insomnia, ECT, computerised CBT for depression and anxiety, ADHD and new drugs in bipolar disorder.

- SIGN (www.sign.ac.uk) has guidance on dementia, bipolar disorder, harmful drinking and alcohol dependence, postnatal depression and puerperal psychosis, attention deficit and hyperkinetic disorders in children and young people, psychosocial interventions in the management of schizophrenia.

- The Royal College of Psychiatrists provides information and guidance on mental health issues: www.rcpsych.ac.uk.

- The PHQ-9 (Patient Health Questionnaire) and HAD (Hospital Anxiety and Depression scale) can be found on www.patient.co.uk.

Statement 14: *Care of People with Learning Disabilities*

There are over 200,000 people living with learning disabilities in the UK. People with learning disabilities have an increased level of associated medical problems and a GP must be aware of the most likely associated conditions and know where to obtain specialist help and advice. GPs must also understand how psychiatric and physical illness may present atypically in patients with sensory, communication and cognitive difficulties. Additional skills of diagnosis and examination are needed to care for patients unable to describe or verbalise their symptoms.

The condensed knowledge

		☑ or score (1–5)
Symptoms	Agitation.	
	Challenging behaviour.	
	Tearfulness.	
	Weight loss and gain.	
	Withdrawal.	
Conditions	Cerebral palsy – especially with severe learning disability.	
	Dermatological problems.	
	Epilepsy – increased incidence and complexity associated with increased severity of learning disability.	
	GI – swallowing problems, reflux oesophagitis, *Helicobacter pylori,* constipation, gastric carcinoma.	
	Obesity – predisposes to other health problems, stigma.	
	Orthopaedic problems – joint contractures, osteoporosis.	
	Psychiatric problems – emotional and behavioural disorders, schizophrenia, bipolar affective disorder, Alzheimer's disease in Down's syndrome.	
	Respiratory problems – chest infections, aspiration pneumonia.	

		☑ or score (1–5)
Conditions	Sensory impairments – hearing and vision disorders, earwax.	
	Sexual and physical abuse.	
Treatment	Hurdles in the delivery of treatment due to difficulties reading instructions and treatment labels.	
	The risks of 'over the counter' prescriptions in some patients who may not fully understand how or why to take treatments but live with a degree of independence.	
	Issues around implementation of interventions – dependency on carers, the difficulties with drug delivery in residential care homes.	
	Difficulties around identifying drug side effects.	
Emergency	In urgent life-threatening cases treatment needs to proceed in the best interests of a person with insufficient capacity to consent.	
Resources	Specialist learning disability teams and non-medical agencies.	
Prevention	Health reviews proposed for people with learning disabilities.	

The condensed skills

		☑ or score (1–5)
Adult learning skills	Addressing barriers to health care for people with learning disabilities including a lack of specialist knowledge and appropriate support services (e.g. behavioural support, psychiatric or neurological assessment services).	
Consultation skills	Maintaining a patient-centred approach while communicating with carers and respecting the patient's autonomy, and also being aware how communication with carers may skew the doctor–patient relationship.	
Time-management skills	Providing more time in the consultation to manage people with learning disabilities more effectively.	

The condensed know-how

	☑ or score (1–5)

The scientific evidence regarding the health needs of people with learning disabilities, in the following areas:

- Untreated, yet treatable, medical conditions
- Untreated specific health issues related to the individual's disability
- A lack of uptake of generic (non-targeted) health promotion.

The difficulties faced by patients with mild learning disabilities, who may need no particular special services, but who may have reading, writing and comprehension difficulties.

Tip: *Arrange an attachment with a community speech and language therapist.*

The difficulties faced by patients with moderate, severe and profound learning disabilities who have special needs for accessing services and need to be identified, monitored and reviewed appropriately.

Tip: *Do a case study on a patient in your practice with learning difficulties and the issues they face.*

The likely conditions associated with learning disability, their common medical problems and where to obtain specialist help and advice.

Tip: *Find out about your local enablement centre and the services they provide.*

Techniques to optimise communication through the use of communication aids, and the impact of the doctor's working environment on patient care (e.g. the measures taken to compensate for sensory impairment).

The particular issues around equitable access to services and information, and maintaining continuity of care in people with learning disabilities.

How psychiatric and physical illness may present atypically in patients with learning disabilities who have sensory, communication and cognitive difficulties.

Tip: *Consider the impact of 'diagnostic overshadowing', when a doctor incorrectly assumes a person's symptoms are due to his or her learning disability rather than an alternative underlying cause.*

How to use additional enquiry, appropriate tests and careful examination in patients unable to describe or verbalise symptoms.

The issues around health promotion in people with learning difficulties.

☑ **or score**
(1–5)

The roles of paid carers, respite care opportunities, day centres, and voluntary and statutory agencies.	
Tip: *Find out who is entitled to Attendance Allowance and Disability Living Allowance.*	
The impact of learning difficulties on family dynamics and the implications for physical, psychological and social morbidity in the patient's carers.	
The particular issues around capacity and consent, and the mechanisms by which these can be determined and enhanced.	
Tip: *Information on this and on the Mental Capacity Act 2005 are available on: www.guardianship.gov.uk.*	
The effects of prejudice and unfair discrimination on people with learning difficulties and the duty of GPs to recognise this within themselves, others and practice systems, and take remedial action.	

The condensed resources

- Directgov provides information for disabled people on employment, financial support, accessibility and rights: www.direct.gov.uk.

- The National Autistic Society offers information for health professionals on diagnosing autism and Asperger's syndrome: www.nas.org.uk.

- The University of Newcastle upon Tyne has an excellent resource on the role of general practitioners in caring for people with learning disability: www.ncl.ac.uk/nnp/teaching/disorders/learning/ld_role.html.

Statement 15.1: *Cardiovascular Problems*

Cardiovascular problems are a major cause of morbidity and mortality in the UK: 50 per cent of 45-year-olds subsequently die from coronary heart disease so management of the risk factors is an essential part of health promotion in general practice. Primary and secondary prevention of cardiovascular disease occurs mainly in primary care and has significant clinical benefit. GPs should be competent at managing cardiovascular emergencies and accurately diagnosing symptoms that may be due to cardiovascular causes.

The condensed knowledge

		☑ or score (1–5)
Symptoms	Ankle swelling.	
	Breathlessness.	
	Chest pain.	
	Collapse.	
	Palpitations and silent arrhythmias.	
	Relating to cerebrovascular disease.	
	Relating to peripheral vascular disease.	
Conditions	Aneurysms (e.g. abdominal aortic aneurysm [AAA], femoral).	
	Arrhythmias (ectopic beats, atrial fibrillation and flutter, ventricular tachycardias, bradyarrhythmias).	
	Cerebrovascular disease (transient ischaemic attack [TIA] and stroke).	
	Coronary heart disease (angina, acute myocardial infarction [MI], cardiac arrest).	
	Heart failure.	
	Hypertension (essential and malignant).	
	Other cardiac disease (cardiomyopathy, valve problems, congenital heart disease).	
	Peripheral vascular disease (arterial and venous).	
	Thromboembolism.	

		☑ or score (1–5)
Investigation	ECG (interpreting and performing).	
	24-hour ambulatory BP.	
	Sphygmomanometry.	
	Venous dopplers and ankle-brachial pressure index (ABPI).	
	Common secondary-care investigations and treatments.	
Treatment	Management of patients at cardiovascular risk, especially blood pressure and lipid management.	
	Chronic disease management of those with established disease.	
Emergencies	Emergency care of MI.	
	Cardiac arrest.	
	Stroke.	
	Critical ischaemia.	
Prevention	The role of health promotion and lifestyle interventions.	
	Management of cardiovascular risk factors both modifiable (BP, lipids, smoking, alcohol, exercise, obesity, diet) and fixed (ethnicity, sex, family history).	
	Management of relevant co-morbidities (e.g. diabetes mellitus, hyperlipidaemia).	

The condensed skills

		☑ or score (1–5)
Consultation skills	Assessing and explaining the risk of cardiovascular problems clearly and effectively in a non-biased manner.	
IM&T skills	Utilising disease registers and data-recording templates for opportunistic and planned monitoring of cardiovascular problems.	

Continued over

		☑ or score (1–5)
Psychomotor skills	Cardiovascular examination.	
	Blood pressure measurement.	
	Calculation of cardiovascular risk.	
	Performing an ECG and basic interpretation.	
	CPR for children and adults.	

The condensed know-how

	☑ or score (1–5)
What to do when a patient presents with a cardiovascular emergency and how geographical distance influences the treatment of cardiovascular emergencies. **Tip:** *Review the emergency drugs box and protocols in your practice and find out how to locate and use the nearest defibrillator.*	
The role of other primary-care health professionals (e.g. practice nurses), cardiologists and other specialists in acute and chronic cardiovascular disease management, including prevention, rehabilitation and palliative care. **Tip:** *Attend a nurse-led chronic disease management (CDM) clinic; ask about your local specialist community services.*	
How to access specialist cardiovascular services, especially rapid-access chest pain clinics, specialist stroke and heart failure services.	
Strategies for the early detection of cardiovascular problems. **Tip:** *Consider the role of 'well-man' and 'well-woman' clinics.*	
The particular issues around non-concordance for preventive cardiovascular medicines and techniques for negotiating management.	
The rationale for restricting certain investigations and treatments (e.g. open-access echocardiography, statin prescribing).	
DVLA guidelines regarding driving according to cardiovascular risks. **Tip:** *Available on the DVLA website (www.dvla.gov.uk/medical/ataglance.aspx).*	
The social and psychological impact of cardiovascular problems on the patient, his or her family, dependants and employers, and on disability and fitness to work. **Tip:** *The British Heart Foundation produces a series of information leaflets for health professionals on this and related issues: www.bhf.org.uk.*	

☑ or score
(1–5)

The cultural significance that people attach to the heart as a 'seat of emotions'.	
The key government policy documents that influence healthcare provision for cardiovascular problems. **Tip:** *Look up the NSFs for coronary heart disease and for older people.*	
The key national guidelines and research findings that influence management of cardiovascular problems (e.g. the Heart Protection Study). **Tip:** *See the full curriculum statement* (*www.rcgp-curriculum.org.uk*).	
The ethical issues relevant to the management of cardiovascular problems (e.g. the consequences of lifestyle choices and issues of age and race).	

The condensed resources

- NICE (www.nice.org.uk) has produced guidelines on atrial fibrillation, chronic heart failure and hypertension.

- SIGN (www.sign.ac.uk) has produced guidelines on hypertension, stable angina, cardiac rehabilitation, secondary prevention of coronary heart disease after MI, lipids and the primary prevention of CHD, diagnosis and treatment of heart failure due to left ventricular systolic dysfunction, management of patients with stroke, and antithrombotic therapy.

- *Joint British Societies JBS2 Guidelines: prevention of cardiovascular disease in clinical practice* (available at: www.library.nhs.uk).

- Royal College of Physicians: *National Clinical Guidelines for Stroke* (www.rcplondon.ac.uk/pubs/books/stroke/stroke_primarycare_2ed.pdf).

- Specific cardiovascular web resources include:

- British Cardiac Society (www.bcs.com)

- British Hypertension Society (www.bhsoc.org)

- Primary Care Cardiovascular Society (www.pccs.org.uk)

- Cardiovascular risk prediction charts can be found in the back of the BNF and at: www.bhsoc.org/resources/prediction_chart.htm.

- National Service Frameworks for coronary heart disease and older people: www.library.nhs.uk/.

Statement 15.2: *Digestive Problems*

Digestive problems are common in general practice and most gut problems are managed in primary care. Dyspepsia and gastro-oesophageal reflux disease (GORD) are particularly common conditions, affecting around a quarter of the population. The prevention and early treatment of colorectal cancer is a priority of the Department of Health, because it is the second most common cause of cancer death.

The condensed knowledge

		☑ or score (1–5)
Symptoms	Abdominal pain.	
	Anorexia and weight loss.	
	Change in bowel habit.	
	Diarrhoea and constipation.	
	Dyspeptic symptoms.	
	Dysphagia.	
	Haematemesis and melaena.	
	Jaundice.	
	Nausea and vomiting.	
	Rectal bleeding.	
	Tenesmus.	
Conditions	Abdominal masses, organomegally and ascites.	
	Acute abdominal conditions.	
	Coeliac disease and other causes of malabsorption.	
	Constipation.	
	Diverticulosis.	
	Gallstones and gallbladder disease.	
	Gastroenteritis.	
	GORD and hiatus hernia.	

		☑ or score (1–5)
Conditions	GI cancers (including their red flags).	
	Tip: *Refer to the NICE guidelines on referral for suspected cancer (www.nice.org.uk).*	
	Hernias (e.g. inguinal, umbilical and periumbilical, femoral, surgical), incarceration and strangulation.	
	Inflammatory bowel disease (e.g. Crohn's and ulcerative colitis).	
	Irritable bowel syndrome (including making a positive diagnosis).	
	Tip: *Review the Rome III criteria for diagnosing functional bowel disorders: www.romecriteria.org.*	
	Non-ulcer dyspepsia, gastritis and peptic ulceration.	
	Chronic liver disease, malignancy and acute liver failure.	
	Poisoning.	
	Perianal disease.	
Investigation	Blood tests (liver function tests [LFTs], amylase).	
	H. pylori testing.	
	Tip: *Find out the pros and cons of the various methods for this.*	
	Coeliac antibody screening.	
	Stool testing including faecal occult bloods.	
	Abdominal ultrasound.	
	Common secondary-care investigations (endoscopy, barium studies, CT, liver biopsy, ERCP, jejunal biopsy).	
Treatment	Primary-care management of the conditions listed in 'symptoms' and 'conditions'.	
	Awareness of secondary-care management of digestive problems (medical and surgical options).	
Emergencies	Acute abdomen.	
	Haematemesis and melaena.	
	Incarcerated/strangulated hernia.	
Prevention	Dietary advice.	
	Smoking cessation and alcohol advice.	

The condensed skills

		☑ or score (1–5)
Consultation skills	Recognising that some patients find digestive problems, particularly lower GI, difficult to discuss openly and may be embarrassed and reluctant to undergo rectal examination.	
	Communicating the effects of psychological stress on the GI tract in a manner the patient can accept.	
Psychomotor skills	Abdominal examination.	
	Rectal examination.	
	Proctoscopy.	

The condensed know-how

	☑ or score (1–5)
How to recognise and respond urgently to red-flag symptoms, which may indicate GI cancer, the indications for urgent referral and the role of rapid-access GI investigations (and how to access them). **Tip:** *Familiarise yourself with the local criteria for two-week wait referrals.*	
The evidence-based approach to managing dyspepsia, including guidelines, red flags, investigations and the role of endoscopy and prescribing.	
Evaluating the arguments for and against a national screening programme for colorectal cancer. **Tip:** *There is a good summary at www.cancerscreening.org.uk/bowel.*	
Resourcing issues: the rationale for restricting upper GI endoscopy in the management of dyspepsia and the need for increased availability of lower GI endoscopy for the management of colorectal cancer.	
Knowing the GI side effects of common medications.	
Recognising the impact of social and cultural diversity, and the importance of health beliefs relating to diet, nutrition and GI function. **Tip:** *The British Nutrition Foundation (www.nutrition.org.uk) offers advice on cultural diversity and diet.*	
Key national guidelines in the area of digestive problems.	

The condensed resources

- NICE (www.nice.org.uk) has guidance on dyspepsia, obesity, nutritional support in adults and referral for suspected cancer.

- SIGN (www.sign.ac.uk) has guidance on oesophageal and gastric cancer, colorectal cancer, and dyspepsia.

- Specific web resources:

  o Primary Care Society for Gastroenterology: www.pcsg.org.uk

  o British Society of Gastroenterology: www.bsg.org.uk.

Statement 15.3: *Drug and Alcohol Problems*

All GPs have a responsibility for providing general medical care to patients who use drugs and can help to identify, and intervene in, drug misuse before it becomes problematic. Drug use is amenable to treatment, using a combination of psychological, social and medical interventions. Substitution treatment (such as methadone) is effective and, if properly administered, results in improvements in social, medical and psychological functioning, and a reduction in criminal behaviour.

GPs must be familiar with ways of identifying excess alcohol consumption. Despite the prevalence of patients presenting with problems relating to heavy alcohol intake, doctors often fail to make the association. GPs should be aware of the morbidity (physical, psychological and social) caused by alcohol and become practised in a technique called 'brief intervention' (see below), which can have a major impact in reducing alcohol consumption in patients.

The condensed knowledge

		☑ or score (1–5)
Symptoms	Opiate misuse (needle tracks, pinpoint pupils, runny nose, drowsiness).	
	Physical manifestations of alcohol problems (accidents, violence, obesity, dyspepsia, erectile dysfunction, fits, foetal alcohol syndrome, liver damage, anaemia, neurological damage).	
	Psychological manifestations of alcohol problems (anxiety, depression, parasuicide).	
	Stimulant misuse (agitation, skin ulceration).	
	Suggestive of cannabis use (red eyes, irritability, anxiety and panic).	
Conditions	Complications of drug use and misuse relating to the drugs themselves, routes of use and the associated lifestyle issues.	
	Chronic liver disease.	
	Hepatitis B and C.	
	HIV.	

		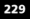 or score (1–5)
Investigation	Urine (and other) tests for drug treatment.	
	Screening tools for alcohol abuse (e.g. CAGE and AUDIT).	
Treatment	Care of drug-abusing patients.	
	Safe prescribing for drug-abusing patients.	
	Brief interventions for excess alcohol use.	
	Management of physical drug and alcohol withdrawal	
Emergencies	Life-threatening drug-related emergencies.	
	Alcohol-related emergencies (fits, delirium and psychosis).	
Prevention	Harm reduction approach.	

The condensed skills

		☑ or score (1–5)
Consultation skills	Establishing and maintaining rapport with patients with drug and alcohol misuse problems, given the chaotic and challenging ways they may use the health service.	
	Enabling patients to recognise that a problem exists, engaging them in delineating their difficulties and deciding on appropriate interventions.	
Reflective and self-awareness skills	Considering issues around stigma and social exclusion, and awareness of your attitudes to these challenging groups of patients.	
Risk assessment skills	Drug use assessment and suicide/self-harm risk assessment.	
	Mental state assessment (and the difficulties involved in assessing an intoxicated patient).	

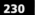

The condensed know-how

	☑ or score (1–5)
The difference between dependent and problematic drug and alcohol use and experimental drug and alcohol use. **Tip:** *Screening tools for the detection of harmful drinking include the Alcohol Use Disorders Identification Test (AUDIT) and CAGE questions.*	
The multifactorial causes of drug misuse and methods for assessing the prevalence of drug and alcohol issue problems in a practice's population.	
The ways patients who use illicit drugs present to services, and the factors that lead to the neglect of health and health care in this group, and steps to counter these. **Tip:** *Review the notes of some of your known drug misusers. Are they receiving optimal physical and mental health care? If not, why not?*	
The role of the wider primary healthcare team, how to access specialists in secondary care and partnerships with the voluntary and criminal justice sector. **Tip:** *Arrange to spend some time with a community addictions worker.*	
The relationship between drug misuse and mental health problems and offending behaviour **Tip:** *Try to arrange some time with a prison doctor, possibly as an attachment or by arranging for him or her to resource a seminar for your learning group.*	
The vulnerability of children whose parents are drug users and how to intervene appropriately.	
How the Misuse of Drugs Act 1971 impacts on health professionals treating drug users. **Tip:** *Find out how to prescribe methadone and subutex, in particular how to arrange for supervised consumption and what to do if a patient reports their 'dog ate the prescription' . . .*	
The political changes that impact on the management of drug misusers.	
Ethical issues around adopting a person-centred approach whilst acknowledging the conflicts between a perceived self-inflicted problem and a right to evidence-based treatment.	

The condensed resources

- Specific web-based resources:
- ○ Substance Misuse Management in General Practice (www. smmgp.org.uk) has produced resources and guidelines on this field and provides information on the RCGP Certificate in the Management of Drug Misuse
- ○ www.drugs.gov.uk is a Home Office website with lots of information
- ○ Talk to Frank (www.talktofrank.com) offers a handy A–Z of slang names for drugs and other advice for the public on drugs
- SIGN (www.sign.ac.uk) has guidance on the management of harmful drinking and alcohol dependence in primary care.

Brief intervention model: 'FRAMES'[30]

F	Feedback	Assessment and evaluation of the problem
R	Responsibility	Emphasising that drinking is by choice
A	Advice	Explicit advice on changing drinking behaviour
M	Menu	Offering alternative goals and strategies
E	Empathy	The role of the counsellor is important
S	Self-efficacy	Instilling optimism that the chosen goals can be achieved

Statement 15.4: *ENT and Facial Problems*

ENT problems, especially ear and throat problems, are common reasons for a visit to the GP. Guidelines for appropriate management of ENT problems are widely available but not widely used. Inappropriate referrals to secondary care increase waiting times, consume resources and can be harmful to patients as early detection of head and neck cancer is vital.

There are 9 million deaf and hard-of-hearing people in the UK, who face considerable communication barriers. The Disability Discrimination Act 1995 gives people with disabilities equal and enforceable rights for access to all areas of life, including health care, and places certain responsibilities on GPs as doctors and employers.

The condensed knowledge

		☑ or score (1–5)
Symptoms	Catarrh.	
	Discharging ear.	
	Dizziness.	
	Dysphagia.	
	Epistaxis.	
	Facial pain (e.g. Bell's palsy, tempero-mandibular pain and trigeminal neuralgia).	
	Facial weakness.	
	Hearing loss and tinnitus.	
	Hoarseness.	
	Neck swellings (e.g. goitre, lymph nodes and other lumps).	
	Otalgia.	
	Sore throat.	
	Speech delay.	
Conditions	Croup.	
	Ear wax.	
	Gingivitis and common dental problems.	
	Nasal polyps.	

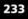 **or score**
(1–5)

Conditions	Otitis externa.	
	Otitis media (suppurative/secretory)	
	Perforated tympanic membrane and cholesteatoma.	
	Pharyngitis and tonsillitis; laryngitis; glandular fever; oral candidiasis, herpes; salivary stones; GORD.	
	Rhinitis (infective and allergic).	
	Sinusitis (infective and allergic).	
	Snoring and sleep apnoea.	
	Suspected head and neck cancer.	
	Trauma (e.g. nasal fracture, haematoma auris).	
	Ulcers (e.g. mouth, pharynx).	
	Unilateral hearing loss in the absence of external ear pathology or obvious cause (e.g. acoustic neuroma).	
	Vertigo and Ménière's disease.	
Investigation	Role of otoscopy	
	Role of tuning-fork tests	
	Awareness of key specialist investigations (pure tone threshold audiogram; speech audiometry, impedance tympanometry, auditory brainstem responses and otoacoustic emissions).	
	Awareness that investigations may delay referral in suspected head and neck cancer.	
Treatment	Watchful waiting and use of delayed prescriptions.	
	Nasal cautery.	
	Fracture of the nose (need manipulation under anaesthetic within two weeks for optimum result).	
Emergencies	Septal haematoma.	
	Epistaxis.	
	Tonsillitis with quinsy.	

Continued over

		☑ or score (1–5)
Emergencies	Otitis externa if extremely blocked or painful; mastoiditis.	
	Foreign bodies (e.g. in ear or nose).	
	Auricular haematoma or perichondritis.	
Prevention	Screening for hearing impairment in adults and children.	
	Awareness of iatrogenic causes of ototoxicity.	

The condensed skills

		☑ or score (1–5)
Communication skills	Communicating effectively with patients with hearing impairment (e.g. remembering to face the patient and speaking clearly so that they can lip read).	
	Dealing effectively with parental concerns regarding common ENT conditions in children (e.g. glue ear, tonsillitis and otitis media).	
Consultation skills	Utilise time as a diagnostic tool (e.g. glue ear), ensuring clear review procedures and safety-netting.	
Negotiation skills	To make referrals appropriately and accurately so people with minor ENT conditions don't compromise the care of those with more serious conditions.	
Psychomotor skills	Otoscopy.	
	Simple nasal cautery.	
	Tuning-fork tests (Weber and Rinne's tests).	
	Throat and neck examination.	

The condensed know-how

	☑ or score (1–5)
An evidence-based approach to antibiotic prescribing for ENT conditions. **Tip:** *Del Mar, Glasziou and colleagues*[31] *have published influential Cochrane reviews on antibiotic prescribing for common ENT conditions, available at www.cochrane.org.*	
Symptoms that fall within the range of normal and require no treatment (e.g. cyclical blocking of nose, senile rhinorrhoea, small neck lymph nodes in well children).	
Indications for appropriate referral to an ENT specialist (e.g. recurrent tonsillitis, ear drum perforations in pars flaccida).	
Issues arising when services are deficient or have long waiting times for ENT surgery (e.g. audiometry, hearing aids, cochlear implants). **Tip:** *What routes of referral can you offer patients who want to be considered for a hearing aid?*	
The role of specialist ENT nurse services and how to access these. **Tip:** *Find out if your local ENT nurses offer urgent aural toilet for otitis externa.*	
The role of self-treatment and how to encourage self-coping strategies where appropriate (e.g. hay fever, nosebleeds, dizziness, tinnitus).	
The red-flag symptoms for head and neck cancer (e.g. hoarseness persisting for more than six weeks, ulceration of oral mucosa persisting for more than three weeks). **Tip:** *Review the NICE guideline on referral for suspected cancer.*	
The ENT presentations of important systemic diseases, e.g. GORD, CVA, AIDS.	
Occupational exposure as a cause of ENT disease (e.g. industrial deafness).	
The national screening programme for hearing loss in neonates. **Tip:** *Find out about the Newborn Hearing Screening Programme at www.nhsp.info.*	
How certain ENT symptoms can indicate psychological distress (e.g. globus – sensation of not swallowing in a patient who can swallow, the 'dizzy' patient who can walk without difficulty).	
The key national guidelines that influence healthcare provision for ENT problems.	

Continued over

The impact of deafness on people's lives and methods to address this, and ways of ensuring that a patient's hearing impairment does not prejudice the communicated information (e.g. using hearing aid loop induction).

Tip: *The Royal National Institute for Deaf People (www.rnid.org.uk) offers advice and support in this area.*

How to provide communications support, such as a BSL/English interpreter or purchasing helpful equipment and putting a prominent reminder on the medical records to alert staff.

Tip: *What strategies does your practice use to ensure hard-of-hearing patients are not disadvantaged?*

The legal implications of the Disability Discrimination Act 1995 for GPs including the need for 'reasonable adjustments' (e.g. allowing more time for appointments or having a display board to announce the next appointment).

The condensed resources

- SIGN (www.sign.ac.uk) has guidance on diagnosis and management of head and neck cancer, diagnosis and management of childhood otitis media in primary care, and management of sore throat and indications for tonsillectomy.

- Evidence-based guidance on managing ENT conditions can be accessed at the Clinical Knowledge Summaries website: http://cks.library.nhs.uk.

Statement 15.5: *Eye Problems*

Around 2 million people in the UK have a sight problem, around 1 million of whom are blind or partially sighted. Eye problems account for 1.5 per cent of GP consultations in the UK with a rate of 50 consultations per 1000 population per year. Eye problems are a significant causes of preventable disabilities and the primary healthcare team plays a key role in the prevention and treatment of eye problems.

The condensed knowledge

		☑ or score (1–5)
Symptoms	Altered vision (e.g. flashes, floaters, distortions, halos).	
	Sticky or itchy eyes.	
	Sudden loss of vision.	
	The painful eye.	
	The red eye.	
Conditions	Disorders of the lids and lacrimal drainage apparatus:	
	• Blepharitis	
	• Stye and chalazion	
	• Entropion and ectropion	
	• Basal cell carcinoma	
	• Naso-lacrimal obstruction and dacryocystitis.	
	External eye disease: sclera, cornea and anterior uvea:	
	• Conjunctivitis (infective and allergic)	
	• Dry-eye syndrome	
	• Episcleritis and scleritis	
	• Corneal ulcers and keratitis	
	• Iritis and uveitis	
	• Orbital cellulitis.	

Continued over

		☑ or score (1–5)
Conditions	Disorders of refraction:	
	• Cataract	
	• Myopia, hypermetropia, astigmatism	
	• Principles of refractive surgery	
	• Problems associated with contact lenses.	
	Disorders of aqueous drainage:	
	• Acute angle closure glaucoma	
	• Primary open angle glaucoma	
	• Secondary glaucomas.	
	Vitreo-retinal disorders:	
	• Flashes and floaters	
	• Macular degeneration	
	• Retinal detachment	
	• Retinoblastoma	
	• Vitreous detachment	
	• Vitreous haemorrhage.	
	Disorders of the optic disc and visual pathways:	
	• Swollen optic disc: recognition and differential diagnosis	
	• Atrophic optic disc: recognition and differential diagnosis	
	• Pathological cupping of the optic disc	
	• Migraine	
	• Transient ischaemic attack (TIA).	
	Eye movement disorders and problems of binocularity:	
	• Amblyopic diplopia	
	• Non-paralytic and paralytic strabismus.	

		☑ or score (1–5)

Investigation	Understanding of appropriate investigations to exclude systemic disease (e.g. erythrocyte sedimentation rate [ESR] for temporal arteritis, chest X-ray [CXR] for sarcoid, etc.).	
	Knowledge of secondary-care investigations and treatment including slit lamp and eye pressure measurement.	
Treatment	Medications including mydriatics, topical anaesthetics, corticosteroids, antibiotics, glaucoma agents.	
	Removal of superficial foreign bodies from the eye.	
Emergencies **Tip:** *Find out how to access emergency eye services in your locality.*	Superficial ocular trauma, including assessment of foreign bodies, abrasions and minor lid lacerations.	
	Arc eye.	
	Severe blunt injury, including hyphaema.	
	Severe orbital injury, including blow-out fracture.	
	Penetrating ocular injury and tissue prolapse.	
	Retained intraocular foreign body.	
	Sudden painless loss of vision (e.g. retinal detachment).	
	Severe intraocular infection.	
	Acute angle closure glaucoma.	
Prevention	Genetics – family history.	
	Co-morbidities especially diabetes and hypertension.	

The condensed skills

		☑ or score (1–5)
Psychomotor skills	Measurement of visual acuity.	
	Pinhole testing.	
	External examination of the eye.	
	Eversion of eyelid.	
	Examination of pupil and assessment of red reflex.	
	Assessment of ocular movements and cover testing.	
	Visual field testing by confrontation.	
	Direct ophthalmoscopy.	
	Colour vision testing.	
	Fluorescein staining of the cornea.	

The condensed know-how

	☑ or score (1–5)
Managing ocular manifestations of neurological disease (e.g. hemianopia, nystagmus, manifestations of pituitary and cerebral tumours).	
Managing ocular manifestations of systemic disease (e.g. diabetic retinopathies, retinal vascular occlusions, amaurosis fugax/transient ischaemic attacks (TIAs), macular diseases, hypertensive retinopathy).	
The organisation of screening for eye problems, how to identify those at risk and how to access services (e.g. diabetic retinopathy, glaucoma, visual acuity testing, squint). **Tip:** *Find out where to direct diabetic patients in need of retinal screening and review the criteria for who should have glaucoma screening.*	
The definition of blindness and partial sightedness, when and how to register a patient, the value of registration and the role of specialist social workers. **Tip:** *Find out the criteria for registration as blind and the procedure for how a patient registers.*	

The psychological and social problems associated with adjustment to chronic visual impairment on the patient and family, the impact of eye problems on disability and fitness to work, the long-term care needs of patients with debilitating eye conditions and the necessary environmental adaptation and use of community resources.

Tip: *Arrange for a visually impaired person to talk to your learning group about his or her experience of daily living.*

Strategies to help a patient maximise visual function through management of disease, preventive care and control of environmental factors, and how to facilitate patient access to sources of support:

• RNIB and talking book services

• Social services; care of the family and financial support

• Local services

• Low vision aids.

Sources of social support for the visually impaired child:

• The 'Statementing' process for children with special educational needs

• Schooling requirements and role of peripatetic teachers

• Career guidance for visually impaired children.

The role of the community optician and appropriate referrals.

The role of other primary care health professionals, optometrists, ophthalmologists, orthoptists, school health services, community eye clinics, and social workers in the care of people with eye problems.

Tip: *Arrange a session in your local eye casualty clinic.*

The DVLA driving regulations for people with visual problems.

Tip: *These can be found at www.dvla.gov.uk/medical/ataglance.aspx.*

The communication issues arising from visual impairment; difficulty receiving written information and accessing healthcare services, and measures to overcome these.

The key national guidelines that influence healthcare provision for eye problems.

Ethical issues around balancing the autonomy of patients with visual problems and public safety (e.g. driving).

The condensed resources

- Royal National Institute for the Blind: www.rnib.org.uk.

- Royal College of Ophthalmologists: www.rcophth.ac.uk.

- NICE (www.nice.org.uk) has provided guidance on the management of retinopathy in Type 2 diabetes.

- The National Service Framework for diabetes is available online at www.library.nhs.uk/.

Statement 15.6: *Metabolic Problems*

The prevalence of obesity and diabetes mellitus is increasing, and these conditions are significant risk factors for medical problems. The management of diabetes, hyperthyroidism and hypothyroidism is primarily carried out in primary care and GPs should be competent in the management of diabetic, thyroid and adrenal emergencies. Hyperuricaemia (gout) is a common cause of morbidity, which is usually diagnosed and managed exclusively in primary care.

The condensed knowledge

		☑ or score (1–5)
Symptoms	Patients with metabolic problems are frequently asymptomatic or have non-specific symptoms, such as tiredness, malaise, weight loss or gain.	
	Diabetes mellitus – tiredness, polydipsia, polyuria, weight loss, infections.	
	Hyperlipidaemia – xanthelasma.	
	Hyperuricaemia – gout.	
	Hypothyroidism – tiredness, weight gain, constipation, hoarse voice, dry skin and hair, menorrhagia.	
	Hyperthyroidism – weight loss, tremor, palpitations, hyperactivity, exophthalmos, double vision.	
	Individual endocrine disorders have typical symptom complexes (e.g. polycystic ovary syndrome [PCOS]).	
Conditions	Adrenal disease (e.g. Cushing's syndrome, hyperaldosteronism, Addison's disease, phaeochromocytoma)	
	Diabetes mellitus – Type 1 and 2.	
	Hyperlipidaemia.	
	Hyperuricaemia.	
	Impaired Glucose Tolerance (and metabolic syndrome).	
	Obesity.	

Continued over

		☑ or score (1–5)
Conditions	Parathyroid disease.	
	Pituitary disease (e.g. prolactinoma, acromegaly, diabetes insipidus).	
	Thyroid disorders – hypothyroidism, hyperthyroidism, goitre, thyroid nodules.	
Investigation	Body mass index calculation.	
	WHO diagnostic criteria for diabetes mellitus. **Tip:** *Find these at www.who.int/diabetes.*	
	Near-patient capillary glucose measurement (including patient self-monitoring).	
	HbA1c and fructosamine to assess glycaemic control.	
	Albumin: creatinine ratio or dipstick for microalbuminuria.	
	Interpret serum electrolyte and urate results.	
	Interpret thyroid function tests and understand their limitations – TSH, T4, free T4, T3, autoantibodies.	
	Interpret lipid profile tests – total cholesterol, HDL, LDL, triglycerides.	
	Visual acuity and retinal photography.	
	Knowledge of secondary-care investigations including the glucose tolerance test, thyroid ultrasound and fine needle aspiration, specialised endocrine tests.	
Treatment	Understand principles of treatment for common conditions managed largely in primary care – obesity, diabetes mellitus, hypothyroidism, hyperlipidaemia, hyperuricaemia.	
	Chronic disease management including specific disease management, systems of care and multidisciplinary teamwork for people with established metabolic problems.	

		☑ or score (1–5)
Treatment	Communication with patients and their families and inter-professional communication both within the PHCT and between primary and secondary care.	
Emergencies	Acute management of diabetic emergencies – hypoglycaemia, hyperglycaemic ketoacidosis and hyperglycaemic hyperosmolar non-ketotic coma.	
	Acute management of thyroid emergencies – myxoedema coma and hyperthyroid crisis.	
	Recognition and primary-care management of Addisonian crisis.	
Prevention	Health promotion activities include dietary modification and exercise advice.	
	Understand when prevention of hyperuricaemia is appropriate, e.g. patients treated for myeloproliferative disorders.	
	Obesity and diabetes mellitus are risk factors for other conditions, so optimal management is preventive.	

The condensed skills

		☑ or score (1–5)
Consultation skills	Ensuring that a patient's weight does not prejudice the information communicated and that the risks of complications are not misleadingly stated (e.g. to coerce a patient into complying with treatment).	
Psychomotor skills	Calculating body mass index.	
	Lower-leg examination for complications of diabetes mellitus.	
	Capillary glucose measurement using a near-patient test.	
	Thyroid examination.	

The condensed know-how

	☑ or score (1–5)

Environmental and genetic factors affecting the prevalence of metabolic problems, diabetes, hypertension and dyslipidaemia.

Tip: *Diabetes is more prevalent in the UK in patients of Asian and Afro-Caribbean origin and hyperuricaemia is more prevalent in prosperous areas and is associated with obesity.*

The local systems of care for metabolic conditions, including the roles of primary and secondary care, shared-care arrangements, multidisciplinary teams and patient involvement.

The role of other primary-care health professionals, such as diabetes nurse specialists, dieticians, district nurses, community matrons, chiropodists and opticians in chronic disease management.

Tip: *Find out how to refer patients to the local diabetes specialist nurses, dieticians and podiatrists.*

The indications for referral to an endocrinologist for management of complex metabolic problems or investigation of certain endocrine disorders.

Risk factors and the role of screening and recognising symptom complexes, as patients with metabolic problems are frequently asymptomatic or have non-specific symptoms.

Tip: *What screening does your practice offer patients at risk of developing Type 2 diabetes?*

Appropriate lifestyle interventions for obesity, diabetes mellitus, hyperlipidaemia and hyperuricaemia.

Tip: *Arrange an attachment with the community dietician.*

Public health interventions and their impact on obesity and diabetes mellitus, and the GP's role in these (e.g. exercise on prescription).

Groups of medication in the management of diabetes (e.g. antiplatelet drugs, angiotensin-converting enzyme inhibitors, angiotensin-II receptor antagonists, and lipid-lowering therapies).

The issues raised by co-morbidity and polypharmacy in diabetes, and strategies to simplify medication regimes and encourage concordance.

Exemptions from prescription charges for patients with metabolic and endocrine conditions.

Tip: *Familiarise yourself with FP92A (Medical Exemption Certificate).*

☑ or score
(1–5)

The psychosocial impact of diabetes and other long-term metabolic problems (e.g. risk of depression, restrictions on employment and driving for diabetes, sexual dysfunction), and the stigma associated with obesity. **Tip:** *Find out about the evidence for ways of screening for depression in chronic disease.*[29]	
How to encourage self-management of metabolic conditions and the role of expert patients.	
The key government policy documents that influence healthcare provision for metabolic problems.	
The key national guidelines that influence healthcare provision for cardiovascular problems (e.g. NICE guidelines, British Hypertension Society Joint Committee Recommendations, National Service Frameworks and quality markers) and the key research findings that influence management of metabolic problems.	

The condensed resources

- The full statement has a list of relevant papers in the 'Further reading' section. The big two studies are DCCT (Diabetes Control and Complications Trial) and UKPDS (UK Prospective Diabetes Study).

- The National Service Framework for diabetes is available at www.library.nhs.uk.

- NICE (www.nice.org.uk) has guidance on Type 1 diabetes and several guidelines on Type 2 diabetes (blood glucose, foot care, blood pressure and lipids, renal disease and retinopathy).

- SIGN (www.sign.ac.uk) has guidelines on the management of diabetes.

- Joint British Societies *JBS2 Guidelines: prevention of cardiovascular disease in clinical practice* (available at www.library.nhs.uk).

- Specific web resources:

- ○ Association of British Clinical Diabetologists: www.diabetologists-abcd.org.uk

- ○ Diabetes UK: www.diabetes.org.uk.

Statement 15.7: *Neurological Problems*

The presentation of a neurological problem may indicate the presence of a disorder confined to a part of the nervous system or may indicate the beginning of a multi-system disease. Symptoms presented to the GP and attributable to a neurological cause may be due to minor self-limiting disease or a more serious problem, so GPs must be able to evaluate the need for any required intervention or referral.

The management of epilepsy in primary care is a key area of general practice and GPs should also be competent in the management of neurological emergencies.

The condensed knowledge

		☑ or score (1–5)
Symptoms	Abnormal movements and chorea.	
	Drowsiness and delirium.	
	Headache.	
	Loss of consciousness and coma.	
	Memory loss and cognitive impairment.	
	Neuropathies.	
	Seizures.	
	Tremor.	
	Vertigo and dizziness (neurological, otological, psychological and cardiovascular causes).	
Conditions	Common causes of headache:	
	• Tension headache	
	• Migraine and cluster headache	
	• Cervical neuralgia, sinusitis and dental pain	
	• Drug rebound headache.	
	Serious causes of headache:	
	• Raised intracranial pressure, tumours	
	• Thunderclap headache (e.g. subarachnoid haemorrhage, enlarging aneurysm or migraine)	
	• Temporal arteritis	

		☑ or score (1–5)

Conditions	● Trigeminal neuralgia	
	● *Herpes zoster.*	
	Amyotrophic lateral sclerosis	
	Brain infections:	
	● Meningitis and encephalitis	
	● Brain abscess	
	● Tuberculosis and HIV.	
	Congenital conditions (e.g. cerebral palsy, spina bifida).	
	Epilepsy.	
	Essential tremor.	
	Genetic conditions (e.g. Huntington's disease).	
	Mononeuropathies including trigeminal neuralgia, Bell's palsy, carpal tunnel syndrome and other nerve entrapments (e.g. ulnar, sciatic and femoral nerves).	
	Multiple sclerosis.	
	Neurological causes of vertigo (e.g. stroke, multiple sclerosis, trauma and concussion, acoustic neuroma, brain tumours).	
	Parkinson's disease.	
	Polyneuropathies including metabolic causes (diabetes, alcohol, B12 and folate, porphyria, uraemia), infectious causes (e.g. Gullain-Barré, postviral, HIV) and drug-induced neuropathy.	
	Speech disorders.	
	Stroke (haemorrhage and infarction).	
	Tip: *Stroke is also covered in statements 9:* Care of Older Adults *and 15.1:* Cardiovascular Problems.	
Investigation	Knowledge of secondary-care investigations and treatment including electroencephalography (EEG), computerised tomography (CT) and magnetic resonance imaging (MRI), nerve conduction studies.	

Continued over

		☑ or score (1–5)
Treatment	Understand principles of treatment for common conditions managed largely in primary care – epilepsy, headaches, vertigo, neuropathic pain, mononeuropathies, essential tremor and Parkinson's disease.	
Emergencies	Acute management of meningitis and meningococcal septicaemia, collapse, loss of consciousness or coma.	
	Understand indications for emergency referral of people with:	
	Stroke	
	Intra-cranial haemorrhage	
	Raised intracranial pressure	
	Temporal arteritis.	
Prevention	Health education and accident prevention advice for people with epilepsy.	
	Vaccination for meningococcal disease. **Tip:** *Check out www.immunisation.nhs.uk.*	
	Understand avoidance of triggers and prophylaxis for migraine.	
	Investigation of people with family history of genetic neurological disease (e.g. berry aneurysm).	

The condensed skills

		☑ or score (1–5)
Consultation skills	Communicating prognosis truthfully and sensitively to patients with incurable/disabling neurological conditions.	
	Sharing uncertainty when required and managing 'difficult' symptoms with multiple causes (e.g. chronic headache, dizziness).	
	Tip: *Discuss strategies for tackling medically unexplained symptoms with your learning group.*	

		☑ or score (1–5)
Psychomotor skills	Examination of cranial nervous system.	
	Examination of peripheral nervous system.	
	Visual acuity.	
	Visual fields.	
	Fundoscopic examination.	

The condensed know-how

	☑ or score (1–5)
The indications for referral to a neurologist for ongoing specialist management (e.g. multiple sclerosis, Parkinson's disease) and for conditions that may be irreversible without early treatment (e.g. ulnar nerve entrapment).	
The functional anatomy of the nervous system as required to aid diagnosis. **Tip:** *This is very relevant to diagnosing common conditions such as carpal tunnel syndrome and sciatica.*	
Epilepsy medication drug interactions and side effects, including contraceptive and pregnancy advice, systems for ensuring regular patient reviews and the issues around compliance. **Tip:** *The higher death rate amongst patients with epilepsy may be related to poor seizure control.*	
The current DVLA medical standards of fitness to drive for neurological conditions, in particular epilepsy. **Tip:** *Find these at www.dvla.gov.uk/medical/ataglance.*	
The impact neurological conditions may have on an individual or family's social and economic wellbeing.	
The key national guidelines that influence healthcare provision for neurological problems. **Tip:** *NICE (www.nice.org.uk) has issued guidelines on epilepsy diagnosis and management.*	
Ethical principles involved when treating an incompetent patient (e.g. unconsciousness), and when treating a patient who is unable to communicate (e.g. dysphasia).	

The condensed resources

- NICE (www.nice.org.uk) has guidelines on epilepsy, head injury, multiple sclerosis and Parkinson's disease.

- SIGN (www.sign.ac.uk) has guidelines on epilepsy and early management of head injury.

- RCP National Clinical Guidelines for Stroke (concise primary-care version): www.rcplondon.ac.uk/pubs/books/stroke/stroke_primarycare_2ed.pdf.

- British Association for the Study of Headache: www.bash.org.uk.

- The National Service Framework for long-term (neurological) conditions is available at: www.library.nhs.uk.

Statement 15.8: *Respiratory Problems*

Respiratory problems, including infections of the upper and lower respiratory tracts, are the most common reason for a consultation in general practice and for emergency medical admission to hospital. There is little evidence to support antibiotic prescribing for everyday upper respiratory infections and antibiotics should be rationed to limit the development of antimicrobial resistance.

Serious respiratory diseases kill one in four people in the UK, and smoking cessation advice is an essential part of health promotion in primary care. The management of asthma and COPD are key competencies for GPs and the full involvement of patients in the management of their respiratory problems is essential.

The condensed knowledge

		☑ or score (1–5)
Symptoms	Breathlessness.	
	Chest pain.	
	Cough.	
	Haemoptysis.	
	Wheeze.	
	Sputum production.	
Conditions	Allergy and anaphylaxis.	
	Aspiration of a foreign body.	
	Asthma.	
	Bronchiolitis.	
	Bronchitis.	
	Chronic cough.	
	Chronic interstitial lung diseases.	
	Chronic obstructive pulmonary disease (COPD).	
	Cystic fibrosis.	
	Epiglottitis, laryngitis and tracheitis.	
	Hypersensitivity pneumonitis.	
	Hypersensitivity pneumonitis.	
	Influenza.	

Continued over

		☑ or score (1–5)
Conditions	Lung cancer.	
	Pneumonia (of any cause).	
	Pneumothorax.	
	Pulmonary embolus.	
	Sore throats and colds.	
	Tonsillitis and peritonsillar abscess.	
	Tuberculosis.	
Investigation	Serial peak flow measurement, including patient diaries.	
	Reversibility testing using peak flow meter.	
	Spirometry.	
	Knowledge of secondary-care investigations and treatment including lung function tests, computerised tomography (CT) and magnetic resonance imaging (MRI).	
Treatment	Understand principles of treatment for common conditions managed largely in primary care – upper and lower respiratory tract infections, asthma, COPD, allergic reactions and anaphylaxis.	
	Inhaler technique for commonly used devices.	
Emergencies **Tip:** *Learn how to use a nebuliser before an emergency!*	Acute management of people presenting with shortness of breath.	
	Acute management of anaphylaxis.	
	Management of exacerbations of asthma and COPD.	
	Understand indications for emergency referral of people with asthma, COPD and anaphylaxis.	
Prevention	Smoking cessation assessment, advice and management.	
	Vaccination against influenza, *Streptococcus pneumoniae, Haemophilus influenzae* B, diphtheria and pertussis.	

		☑ or score (1–5)
Prevention	Health education advice and patient self-management plans for people with asthma and COPD.	
	Understand avoidance of triggers and prophylaxis for allergic conditions.	
	Investigation of people with family history of genetic respiratory disease, e.g. cystic fibrosis.	

The condensed skills

		☑ or score (1–5)
Consultation skills	Negotiating a self-management plan for asthma in partnership with the patient and sensitively informing patients with incurable or disabling respiratory conditions of their prognosis.	
Counselling skills	Giving effective smoking cessation advice and ensuring the doctor–patient relationship is enhanced by this process.	
IM&T skills	Using disease registers and data-recording templates effectively for opportunistic and planned monitoring of respiratory problems, and to ensure continuity of care.	
Psychomotor skills	Peak flow measurement technique using child and adult meters, and accurately interpreting the results.	
	Using peak flow diaries and evaluating the results.	
	Demonstrating and assessing technique for using common inhaler types.	
	Using a hand-held spirometer and interpreting the results.	

The condensed know-how

	☑ or score (1–5)
The role of self-management in respiratory conditions (URTI, asthma).	
The evidence-based approach to antibiotic prescribing for respiratory infections.	
The causes of breathlessness, including coexisting causes (e.g. simultaneous cardiac and respiratory disease) and optimum management for these.	
The role of serial peak flow measurement, reversibility testing and spirometry in the diagnosis of asthma and COPD. **Tip:** *Consider which patients should be screened for COPD (e.g. smoking history, industrial exposure).*	
Guidelines for the emergency management and admission of patients with an acute exacerbation of asthma. **Tip:** *A brief summary of these can be found in the BNF at the start of Section 3 (Respiratory System).*	
The alarm symptoms for lung cancer and indications for urgent investigation and referral to specialist services. **Tip:** *Review the NICE guidelines on referral for suspected cancer (www.nice.org.uk).*	
The role of other primary-care health professionals, such as practice nurses, district nurses and physiotherapists, in chronic respiratory disease management and pulmonary rehabilitation.	
Indications for home oxygen therapy and nebulisers, how to evaluate patients' requirements for these, and safety issues when prescribing home oxygen. **Tip:** *Find out about the practicalities of prescribing and delivering home oxygen and completing a 'HOOF' (Home Oxygen Order Form).*	
Common patient health beliefs regarding smoking and ways to reinforce, modify or challenge these beliefs as appropriate.	
The prevalence of respiratory problems in the community and the current population trends in the prevalence of allergic and respiratory conditions, and particular groups of patients at higher risk of acquiring a respiratory infection.	
Occupational exposure as a cause of respiratory disease (e.g. COPD).	

☑ or score
(1–5)

Disability suffered by people with chronic respiratory problems and its psychosocial impact on the patient, family and society.

Tip: *Look into the local pulmonary rehabilitation service.*

How a GP's personal opinion regarding smoking may influence management decisions for people with respiratory problems.

The key national guidelines that influence healthcare provision for respiratory problems (e.g. the BTS/SIGN guidelines on asthma management, the NICE guidelines on COPD management).

The condensed resources

- NICE (www.nice.org.uk) has guidelines on chronic obstructive pulmonary disease, lung cancer, smoking cessation and TB.

- SIGN (www.sign.ac.uk) has guidelines on asthma (joint with the British Thoracic Society), obstructive sleep apnoea and management of lower respiratory tract infection in adults in the community.

- The British Thoracic Society (www.brit-thoracic.org.uk) has lots of guidelines pertinent to primary care, including asthma (joint with SIGN), COPD, cough, lung cancer, pneumonia, suspected pulmonary embolism, pulmonary rehabilitation, sleep apnoea and smoking cessation.

- The General Practice Airways Group is primary-care practitioners with a special interest in chest medicine: www.gpiag.org.

Statement 15.9: *Rheumatology and Conditions of the Musculoskeletal System (including Trauma)*

Musculoskeletal conditions are common, accounting for 15–20 per cent of GP consultations. They lead to significant disability and have huge resource implications from causing incapacity to work. For many GPs in training, experience of musculoskeletal problems has been limited, and appropriate management and referral to allied health professionals, complementary therapists and secondary care is a key competency.

The condensed knowledge

		☑ or score (1–5)
Symptoms	Inflammation – pain, swelling, redness, warmth.	
	Injuries – cuts, bruises, burns, wounds, sprains, fractures.	
	Loss of function – weakness, restricted movement, deformity and disability.	
	Systemic manifestations – rashes, tiredness, nerve compression, etc.	
Conditions	Acute arthropathies.	
	Back/neck pain – acute.	
	Back/neck pain – chronic.	
	Chronic disability.	
	Chronic inflammatory arthropathies.	
	Common injuries and sprains.	
	Fibromyalgia and allied syndromes.	
	Fractures.	
	Head injury.	
	Internal injuries of the chest, abdomen and pelvis.	
	Knee pain (e.g. ligamentous injuries, cartilage tears, arthritis).	
	Osteoarthritis.	
	Osteoporosis.	

		☑ or score (1–5)
Conditions	Pain management.	
	Polymyalgia rheumatica and allied conditions.	
	Shoulder disorders (e.g. rotator cuff tears, capsulitis, impingement).	
	Soft-tissue disorders (e.g. bursitis, synovitis, tendonitis).	
	Awareness of rarer musculoskeletal and rheumatological diseases.	
Investigation	Indications for plain radiography, ultrasound, CT and MR scan including the use of tools such as the 'Ottawa Rules'. **Tip:** *www.gp-training.net/rheum/ottawa.htm is a useful guide to the Ottawa Ankle Rules.*	
	General rules of X-ray interpretation.	
	Implications of 'misses' on X-rays and common errors.	
	Indications for additional investigations, for example blood tests.	
Treatment	Understand the principles of treatment for common conditions managed largely in primary care including the use and monitoring of NSAIDs and disease-modifying drugs.	
	Knowledge of when joint injections and aspirations are appropriate in general practice, and the ability to perform when appropriate, e.g. shoulder and knee joints and injections for tennis and golfer's elbow.	
	The roles of allied health professionals (nursing, physiotherapy, chiropody, podiatry, occupational therapy, counselling and psychological services).	
	Chronic disease management principles, including systems of care, multidisciplinary teamwork and shared-care arrangements.	

Continued over

		☑ or score (1–5)
Emergencies	The initial management of the patient who has been burnt.	
	Tip: *Look at http://cks.library.nhs.uk for an evidence-based guideline on managing burns in primary care.*	
	Awareness of the safety of the patient, the scene of the incident and medical staff.	
	Awareness of how to summon help in an emergency.	
	Competency in basic life support (adult and paediatric), the use of simple airway adjuncts (for example oropharyngeal airway and pocket mask) and the safe use of a defibrillator.	
	Competency in stopping haemorrhage.	
	Competency in reducing pain by the use of analgesia or other methods.	
	Awareness of the principles of major incident management.	
	Referrals requiring emergency action to save life or prevent serious long-term sequelae.	
Prevention	Advise regarding appropriate levels of exercise.	
	Heath promotion regarding accident prevention.	

The condensed skills

		☑ or score (1–5)
Communication skills	Giving health information effectively to patients and communicating truthfully and sensitively to those for whom therapeutic options have been exhausted.	
Consultation skills	Addressing the psychological effects of trauma (e.g. post-traumatic stress disorder), avoiding investigations or treatments unlikely to alter outcomes (e.g. inappropriate back imaging) and prioritising referrals appropriately.	

		☑ or score (1–5)
Psychomotor skills	Examination of the following areas:	
	● The neck and back	
	● The shoulder, elbow, wrist and hand	
	● The hip, knee and ankle.	
	Suturing techniques and simple dressings.	

The condensed know-how

	☑ or score (1–5)
The epidemiology of musculoskeletal disorders at all ages, and how this informs a differential diagnosis, the aetiology and natural history of common and important musculoskeletal conditions.	
The role of blood tests and imaging methods in diagnosis, how to interpret them and how they influence management. **Tip:** *Audit the regular monitoring of blood tests of patients taking disease-modifying drugs (DMARDS) – known as 'near-patient testing'.*	
The roles of the primary healthcare team, allied health professionals, complementary therapists and secondary care (e.g. in shared-care protocols), and how to refer appropriately to the most appropriate healthcare practitioner (e.g. GPs with Special Interests [GPwSI], physiotherapist, podiatrist, osteopath, chiropractor, orthopaedic surgeon, and rheumatologist), shared-care arrangements, multidisciplinary teams and expert-patient involvement. **Tip:** *Try to spend time shadowing a variety of these practitioners.*	
The urgent management of trauma (e.g. basic life support, control of haemorrhage, summoning help) and how geographical distance influences the treatment of trauma in a primary-care setting.	
How the mechanism of an injury may inform the diagnosis.	
How to distinguish inflammatory from non-inflammatory conditions.	
Assessment and management of the psychological factors causing or contributing to musculoskeletal symptoms.	
Iatrogenic problems caused by the treatment of musculoskeletal disorders (e.g. GI bleeds, osteoporosis, coronary heart disease) and the prevention of these. **Tip:** *Find out what systems your practice has in place to reduce methotrexate prescribing errors.*	

Continued over

The GP's role in the assessment of musculoskeletal disability and mobility.

Tip: *Find out how patients apply for a disabled parking badge and the GP's role in the process.*

How to access patient educational resources, e.g. educational material such as the ARC information leaflets and support groups.

Tip: *Arthritis Research Campaign website: www.arc.org.uk.*

Self-help strategies to empower the patient, e.g. self-treatment measures, the expert-patient programme (DH), Challenging Arthritis Programme (Arthritis Care) and local exercise programmes.

Tip: *The Expert Patients Programme (www.expertpatients.nhs.uk) provides opportunities for people with long-term chronic conditions to develop skills to better manage their condition.*

The wider resource implications of incapacity for work due to musculoskeletal conditions.

Tip: *The Department for Work and Pensions website contains a guide for medical practitioners on sickness certification and commonly asked questions: www.dwp.gov.uk/medical.*

Indications for referral to complementary medical services, considering that many services have limited NHS availability or are only available privately.

The role of occupation in musculoskeletal disease (e.g. repetitive strain injury) and the likely prognosis in relation to the occupation.

The key national guidelines for musculoskeletal problems.

The condensed resources

- NICE (www.nice.org.uk) has guidelines on falls, head injury, and post-traumatic stress disorder.

- SIGN (www.sign.ac.uk) has guidelines on management of osteoporosis, prevention and management of hip fracture in older people, and management of early rheumatoid arthritis.

- Primary Care Rheumatology Society: www.pcrsociety.org.uk.

- National Osteoporosis Society: www.nos.org.uk.

- Arthritis Research Campaign offers information for health professionals and patients: www.arc.org.uk.

- The Disabled Living Foundation website (www.dlf.org.uk) has a section for health professionals and includes useful advice on disability products and disabled equipment for older and disabled people, their carers and families.

Statement 15.10: *Skin Problems*

Approximately a quarter of the population are affected by skin problems that would, if they received treatment, benefit from medical care. Most skin problems are managed in primary care, yet traditionally undergraduate and postgraduate training in skin problems has been very limited. Skin disfigurement causes considerable psychological distress and the effective diagnosis and urgent referral of potential melanomas can save lives.

The condensed knowledge

		☑ or score (1–5)
Symptoms	Bruising or purpura.	
	Hair loss.	
	Itch (also known as pruritus).	
	Lumps in and under the skin.	
	Nail problems.	
	Photosensitivity and 'the red face'.	
	Pigmented skin lesions.	
	Rashes.	
	Signs of infections of the skin.	
Conditions	Acne and rosacea.	
	Drug eruptions.	
	Eczema.	
	Generalised pruritus.	
	Hair and nail disorders.	
	Infections of the skin (bacterial, viral and fungal).	
	Infestations including scabies and head lice.	
	Ingrowing toenails.	
	Leg ulcers and lymphoedema.	
	Psoriasis.	
	Skin tumours (benign and malignant).	
	Urticaria.	
	Vasculitis.	

or score
(1–5)

Conditions	Awareness of other less common skin conditions such as the bullous disorders, lichen planus, vitiligo, photosensitivity, pemphigus, pemphigoid, discoid lupus, granuloma annulare and lichen sclerosus.	
Investigation	Ability to take specimens for mycology from skin, hair and nail.	
	Basic interpretation of histology reports.	
	Skin biopsy.	
Treatment	Those commonly used in primary care (including an awareness of appropriate quantities to be prescribed and how to apply them). **Tip:** *Familiarise yourself with the topical steroids potency ladder and fingertip units.*	
	Principles of protective care (sun care, occupational health and hand care).	
	An awareness of specialised treatments, such as retinoids, ciclosporin, phototherapy and methotrexate.	
	The indications for and the skills to perform curettage, cautery and cryosurgery.	
Emergency	Angioedema and anaphylaxis.	
	Meningococcal sepsis.	
	Disseminated herpes simplex.	
	Erythroderma.	
	Pustular psoriasis.	
	Severe nodulocystic acne.	
	Toxic epidermal necrolysis.	
	Stevens–Johnson syndrome.	
	Necrotising fasciitis.	
Prevention	Sun exposure.	
	Fixed factors: family history and genetics (how genetic factors influence the inheritance of common diseases such as psoriasis and atopic eczema).	
	Occupation and care of the hands.	

The condensed skills

		☑ or score (1–5)
Consultation skills	Ensuring that skin problems are not dismissed as trivial and patients with chronic skin problems are helped to manage the effects of disfigurement.	
	Taking a detailed history of change and assessing risk factors in a patient reporting change in a pigmented skin lesion.	
Psychomotor skills	Curettage, cautery and cryosurgery.	
	Skin biopsy.	
	Specimens for mycology from skin, hair and nail.	

The condensed know-how

	☑ or score (1–5)
The promotion of skin wellbeing, including sun protection, occupational health advice and hand care.	
Criteria for referral to specialist services, especially to rapid-access pigmented lesion (sometimes called skin cancer, mole or melanoma) clinics.	
The role of self-management in skin conditions (e.g. eczema and psoriasis).	
The role of other primary-care team members (e.g. district and tissue viability nurses) and shared-care arrangements in the management of many skin problems, e.g. pigmented lesions, ulcers, psoriasis.	
The side effects of common medicines used to prevent and treat other conditions that may cause skin problems. **Tip:** *Look up the skin complaints associated with commonly used drugs such as amiodarone, beta-blockers, lithium, steroids (inhaled, systemic and topical), retinoids and tetracyclines.*	
The rationale for restricting certain investigations and treatments in the management of skin problems (e.g. patch testing, prescribing of retinoids, access to phototherapy). **Tip:** *Find out your local referral restrictions for cosmetic skin problems, and consider the difficulties these raise.*	

The social and psychological impact of skin problems on quality of life; the effects of disfigurement or sleep deprivation as a result of itching.

Tip: *The British Red Cross Skin Camouflage Service offers a free simple skin camouflage service to assist people with a disfigurement.*

Assessing occupational risk in the aetiology of skin disease.

Guidelines and procedures for ensuring informed consent is obtained for procedures (e.g. minor surgery).

The key national guidelines that influence healthcare provision for skin problems (e.g. the NHS cancer plan 2000).

The condensed resources

- SIGN (www.sign.ac.uk) has a guideline for melanoma.
- British Association of Dermatologists: www.bad.org.uk.
- Primary Care Dermatology Society: www.pcds.org.uk.
- Specific web-based resources:
- ○ DermIS online dermatology atlas: www.dermis.net
- ○ DermNet NZ: www.dermnetnz.org
- ○ Google Images is useful for quickly locating pictures of skin conditions: www.google.co.uk.

Statement 15.X: *The Rest of General Practice*

The RCGP Curriculum for Specialty Training for General Practice is a competency-based document, describing the core knowledge and skills required to be a GP (as described in Chapter 6, 'The core competences'). One of the key competencies a GP must acquire is 'managing primary contact with patients and dealing with unselected problems'. This includes being able to deal with virtually every kind of problem and every kind of patient that walks through the surgery door.

Although the curriculum is a large and comprehensive document, it is inevitable that some clinical topics are not mentioned explicitly. This does not mean such topics should not be learned or taught if appropriate; learning to be a successful GP requires mastering the skills required to become a self-directed and needs-based learner, and this involves learning whatever needs to be learned to competently perform the role of a GP.

In this condensed statement, we have included a number of topics that are not explicitly covered by their own curriculum statement. This includes topics described in the syllabus for the new MRCGP (see Chapter 5, 'Succeeding at the new MRCGP') and which may be assessed in the new MRCGP assessments. GP learners and educators should consider whether they need to incorporate these into their learning and teaching plans when preparing for the new MRCGP assessments.

Clinical topics not currently covered by a curriculum statement:

		☑ or score (1–5)
Haematology	Anaemia.	
	Bleeding disorders.	
	Clotting disorders and VTE/DVT.	
	Haematological investigations (e.g. FBC, film, ESR, D-dimers, B12/folate, haematinics).	
	Lymphadenopathy.	
	Lymphoproliferative disorders.	
	Myelodysplasia and myeloproliferative disorders.	
	Paraproteinaemias and myeloma.	
	Post-splenectomy prophylaxis.	

		☑ or score (1–5)
Haematology	Red-cell disorders and haemolysis.	
	Warfarin (initiation and monitoring).	

		☑ or score (1–5)
Renal problems	Acute renal failure.	
	Haematuria (and microhaematuria).	
	Glomerulonephritis.	
	Nephrotic syndrome.	
	Proteinuria.	
	Pyelonephritis and UTI.	
	Renal and bladder stones.	
	Renal replacement therapy (primary-care issues relating to dialysis and transplantation).	
	Renal function test interpretation and monitoring (e.g. U+E, creatinine, eGFR, 24-hour urinary collection tests, microalbuminaemia, proteinuria).	
	Renal impairment and chronic renal failure.	
	Renal tract imaging (e.g. CT, USS).	
	Urinary tract malignancies (e.g. renal, bladder).	

Tip: *Lower urinary tract problems (e.g. cystitis, urinary incontinence and retention) are covered in condensed statements 10.1:* Women's Health *and 10.2:* Men's Health.

Tip: *The Renal Association provides useful information for GPs on chronic renal conditions (www.renal.org).*

☑ **or score**
(1–5)

Infectious diseases	Bacterial infections not covered elsewhere in the curriculum (e.g. brucellosis, diphtheria, endocarditis, erysipelas staphylococcus, streptococcus, legionella, listeria, Lyme disease, psittacosis, tetanus, treponema).	
	Food poisoning (e.g. botulism, campylobacter, salmonella, *E. coli*, rotavirus)	
	Hospital-acquired infections (e.g. MRSA and clostridium).	
	Influenza vaccination campaigns and management of high-risk groups; flu pandemic planning.	
	Notifiable diseases and role of public health in infectious disease control and contact tracing.	
	Parasitic and protozoal infections (e.g. head lice, threadworms, toxoplasmosis, scabies).	
	Postviral fatigue syndrome.	
	Pyrexia of unknown origin.	
	Routine immunisation schedules and issues around vaccination (e.g. MMR, BCG, pneumovax).	
	Systemic fungal infections (e.g. aspergillosis, oral candidiasis, pityriasis).	
	Travel advice and vaccinations; malaria prophylaxis.	
	Tropical diseases (e.g. malaria, amoebic dysentery, giardiasis), traveller's diarrhoea.	
	Viral infections not covered elsewhere in the curriculum (e.g. CMV, hepatitis A, herpes simplex, herpes zoster, HIV, influenza, infectious mononucleosis, hand, foot and mouth, measles, mumps, parvovirus, rubella, varicella).	

		☑ or score (1–5)
Surgery	Evaluating a patient's fitness for surgery.	
	Optimising a patient's fitness for surgery.	
	Managing common post-surgical complications after discharge.	
	Routine wound care and healing.	
	Recovery, rehabilitation and return to work after surgery.	

		☑ or score (1–5)
Miscellaneous	Medically unexplained symptoms.	
	Chronic fatigue syndrome.	
	Off legs.	
	Common occupational health issues.	

Other clinical topics _you_ have identified a need to learn:

		☑ or score (1–5)

References

1 Helman CG. Disease versus illness in general practice *Journal of the Royal College of General Practice* 1981; **31**: 548–62.

2 Rosenstock I. *Historical Origins of the Health Belief Model.* Health Education Monographs. Vol. 2 No. 4, 1974.

3 Pendleton D, Schofield T, Tate P, Havelock P. *The Consultation: an approach to learning and teaching* Oxford: Oxford University Press, 1984.

4 Caldicott Committee, DoH. *Report on the Review of Patient-Identifiable Information* London: Department of Health, 1997 (available at: www.dh.gov.uk).

5 General Medical Council. *Good Medical Practice* London: General Medical Council, 2006 (available at: www.gmc-uk.org).

6 Stott N C and Davis R H. The exceptional potential in each primary care consultation *Journal of the Royal College of General Practitioners* 1979; **29**: 201–5.

7 Neighbour R. *The Inner Consultation* Lancaster: MTP, 1987.

8 Tuckett D, Boulton M, Olson C, Williams A. *Meetings between Experts* London: Tavistock Publications, 1985.

9 Stewart M, Brown JB, Weston WW, McWhinney IR, McWilliam CL, Freeman T. Patient-centred medicine, in *Transforming the Clinical Method* (2nd edn), Abingdon: Radcliffe Medical Press Ltd, 2003.

10 Kurtz SM and Silverman JD. The Calgary–Cambridge observation guides: an aid to defining the curriculum and organizing the teaching in communication training programmes *Medical Education* 1996; **30**: 83–9.

11 Kurtz SM, Silverman JD, Draper J. *Teaching and Learning Communication Skills in Medicine* Oxford: Radcliffe Medical Press, 1998.

12 Information about PDSA cycles can be found on the NHS Modernisation Agency website: www.wise.nhs.uk [accessed June 2007].

13 Royal College of General Practitioners/General Practitioners Committee. *Good Medical Practice for General Practitioners* London: RCGP, 2002.

14 Acheson D. *Inequalities in Health: report of an independent inquiry* London: HMSO, 1998.

15 www.peterhoney.com [accessed June 2007].

16 Crockett P and Hull A. How to negotiate effectively *BMJ Careers* 15 February; **326**: s49–50.

17 Maslow AH. *Motivation and Personality* New York: Harper & Row, 1954.

18 McClelland DC. *Human Motivation* San Francisco: Scott Foresman, 1985.

19 Belbin RM. *Management Teams: why they succeed or fail* Oxford: Butterworth-Heinemann, 1981.

20 Wilson JMG and Junger G. *Principles and Practice of Screening for Disease* Geneva: WHO, 1968.

21 Hall D and Elliman D. *Health for All Children* (4th edn) Oxford: Oxford University Press, 2003.

22 DiClemente C C, Prochaska J O, Fairhurst S K, Velicer W F, *et al*. The process of smoking cessation: an analysis of precontemplation, contemplation, and preparation stages of change *Journal of Consulting and Clinical Psychology* 1991; **59**: 295–304.

23 Tudor Hart J. The inverse care law *Lancet* 1971; **i**: 405–12.

24 Medical Protection Society. *Case Reports* Vol. 13: 3, August 2005.

25 Department of Health. *Best Practice Guidance for Doctors and Other Health Professionals on the Provision of Advice and Treatment to Young People under 16 on Contraception, Sexual and Reproductive Health* London: DoH, 2004 [available at: www.dh.gov.uk].

26 Fick D M, Cooper J W, Wade W E, Waller J L, *et al*. Updating the Beers criteria for potentially inappropriate medication use in older adults: results of a US consensus panel of experts *Archives of Internal Medicine* 2003; **163**: 2716–24.

27 Scottish Executive. *Adding Life to Years* Edinburgh: Scottish Executive, 2001.

28 RCGP curriculum statement 10.2: *Men's Health* London: RCGP, 2006.

29 Arroll B, Khin N, Kerse N. Screening for depression in primary care with two verbally asked questions: cross sectional study *British Medical Journal* 2003; **327**: 1144–6.

30 Miller W R and Sanchez V C. Motivating young adults for treatment and lifestyle change. In: G Howard (ed.). *Issues in Alcohol Use and Misuse in Young Adults* Notre Dame: University of Notre Dame Press, 1993.

31 Glasziou P P, Del Mar C B, Sanders S L. Antibiotics for acute otitis media in children *Cochrane Database of Systematic Reviews*, 2004, Issue 1. Art. No.: CD000219. DOI: 10.1002/14651858.CD000219.pub2.

Appendix 1
Curriculum domains grid for planning learning activities

Learning Objective(s):

Essential Application Features

Core Competences	Contextual	Attitudinal	Scientific
1. Primary care management	What: When:	What: When:	What: When:
2. Person-centred care	What: When:	What: When:	What: When:
3. Specific problem-solving skills	What: When:	What: When:	What: When:
4. A comprehensive approach	What: When:	What: When:	What: When:
5. Community orientation	What: When:	What: When:	What: When:
6. A holistic approach	What: When:	What: When:	What: When:

Appendix 2
Common GP topics mapped to the relevant curriculum statements

The following table lists GP topics commonly learned or taught in educational and training activities. These have been mapped to their relevant curriculum statements, which have all been summarised in Chapter 7, 'The essential knowledge'.

Statement 1: *Being a General Practitioner* is the core curriculum statement and can be used as a wide-ranging resource for most educational activities in general practice. As it is so wide-ranging, it is not included in the following table. The generic competencies and expertise required of a GP are explored in depth in Chapter 6, 'The core competences'.

Clinical topics where the relevant curriculum statement is very obvious have not been included (e.g. skin rashes are covered by statement 15.10: *Skin Problems*).

Common GP topics	Relevant curriculum statement(s)
Abdominal pain (chronic)	15.2 *Digestive Problems* 8 *Care of Children and Young People*
Accounts and book-keeping	4.1 *Management in Primary Care*
Acute abdomen	7 *Care of Acutely Ill People* 15.2 *Digestive Problems*
Adult learning skills	3.7 *Teaching, Mentoring and Clinical Supervision*
Alcohol problems	15.3 *Drug and Alcohol Problems*
Anaemia	15.X *The Rest of General Practice**
Antenatal care	10.1 *Women's Health*
Antenatal testing	6 *Genetics in Primary Care* 10.1 *Women's Health*
Anxiety and panic attacks	13 *Care of People with Mental Health Problems*
Appointment systems	4.1 *Management in Primary Care*
Arthritis	15.9 *Rheumatology and Conditions of the Musculoskeletal System (including Trauma)*
Asthma	7 *Care of Acutely Ill People* 8 *Care of Children and Young People* 15.8 *Respiratory Problems*

Prostate disorders	10.2	*Men's Health*
Protocols and guidelines	3.5	*Evidence-Based Practice*
Psychiatric emergencies	7	*Care of Acutely Ill People*
	13	*Care of People with Mental Health Problems*
Psychosexual problems	10.1	*Women's Health*
	10.2	*Men's Health*
	11	*Sexual Health*
Quality assurance	3.1	*Clinical Governance*
	4.1	*Management in Primary Care*
Record keeping	4.2	*Information Management and Technology*
Red eye	15.5	*Eye Problems*
Referral systems	2	*The General Practice Consultation*
	12	*Care of People with Cancer and Palliative Care*
Relationship difficulties	13	*Care of People with Mental Health Problems*
Relationships with colleagues	3.1	*Clinical Governance*
Relationships with patients	2	*The General Practice Consultation*
Renal problems	10.1	*Women's Health*
	10.2	*Men's Health*
	15.X	*The Rest of General Practice**
Repeat prescriptions	3.2	*Patient Safety*
Research	3.6	*Research and Academic Activity*
Residential and nursing care	9	*Care of Older Adults*
Respect for patients' dignity	3.4	*Promoting Equality and Valuing Diversity*
Resuscitation and BLS	7	*Care of Acutely Ill People*
Screening programmes	5	*Healthy People*
Services for the disabled	9	*Care of Older Adults*
	13	*Care of People with Mental Health Problems*
Sickness certification	2	*The General Practice Consultation*
Significant event analysis	3.2	*Patient Safety*
Smoking	5	*Healthy People*
Sports injuries	15.9	*Rheumatology and Conditions of the Musculoskeletal System (including Trauma)*
Statistics	3.5	*Evidence-Based Practice*
Sterilisation	10.1	*Women's Health*
	10.2	*Men's Health*
	11	*Sexual Health*
Stroke	9	*Care of Older Adults*
	15.1	*Cardiovascular Problems*
	15.7	*Neurological Problems*

Suicide and deliberate self-harm	13	*Care of People with Mental Health Problems*
Surgery	15.X	*The Rest of General Practice**
Teaching skills	3.7	*Teaching, Mentoring and Clinical Supervision*
Teenage health care	8	*Care of Children and Young People*
	11	*Sexual Health*
	15.3	*Drug and Alcohol Problems*
Telephone consultations	2	*The General Practice Consultation*
	3.2	*Patient Safety*
Terminal care	12	*Care of People with Cancer and Palliative Care*
Termination of pregnancy	10.1	*Women's Health*
	11	*Sexual Health*
Thyroid disease	15.6	*Metabolic Problems*
Time management	2	*The General Practice Consultation*
Travel advice and vaccinations	15.X	*The Rest of General Practice**
Uncertainty, dealing with	2	*The General Practice Consultation*
Urinary disorders	10.1	*Women's Health*
	10.2	*Men's Health*
Use of time as a diagnostic tool	2	*The General Practice Consultation*
Venous thrombosis	15.1	*Cardiovascular Problems*
Vertigo and dizziness	15.4	*ENT and Facial Problems*
	15.7	*Neurological Problems*
Violence	3.2	*Patient Safety*
	10.1	*Women's Health*
	10.2	*Men's Health*
Visual impairment and blindness	15.5	*Eye Problems*
Warfarin monitoring	15.X	*The Rest of General Practice**
Work–life balance	3.1	*Clinical Governance*
X-rays and imaging services	3.5	*Evidence-Based Practice*

*15.X: *The Rest of General Practice* is not an official curriculum statement. It was created in *The Condensed Curriculum Guide* to contain topics identified in the new MRCGP syllabus that are not explicitly described in an existing curriculum statement.

Index

NB Entries in *italic* denote published materials or curriculum statements